T.J. Priestman

Cancer Chemotherapy: an Introduction

Third Edition

Springer-Verlag
London Berlin Heidelberg New York
Paris Tokyo

T.J. Priestman MD, FRCP, FRCR

Consultant Radiotherapist and Clinical Oncologist, Queen
Elizabeth Hospital, Edgbaston, Birmingham B15 2TH, U.K.

ISBN 3–540–19551–3 Springer Verlag Berlin Heidelberg New York
ISBN 0–387–19551–3 Springer Verlag New York Berlin Heidelberg
(ISBN 0 9505545 1 0 second edition)

British Library Cataloguing in Publication Data
Priestman, Terry J. (Terry James)
   Cancer chemotherapy. – 3rd ed.
   1. Man. Cancer. Drug therapy
   I. Title
   616.99'4061
   ISBN 3–540–19551–3

Library of Congress Cataloging-in-Publication Data
Priestman, Terry J.
   Cancer chemotherapy.
   Bibliography: p.
   Includes index.
   1. Cancer–Chemotherapy. I. Title. [DNLM: 1. Anti-
neoplastic Agents–therapeutic use. 2. Neoplasma–drug
therapy. QZ 267 P949c]
RC271.C5P74 1989   616.99'4061   89–5999
ISBN 0–387–19551–3 (U.S.)

©Springer-Verlag Berlin Heidelberg 1989
First published 1977 by Montedison Pharmaceuticals Ltd.
Revised edition 1980 published by Farmitalia Carlo Erba Ltd.
Printed in Great Britain

The use of registered names, trademarks etc. in this publication does not imply,
even in the absence of a specific statement, that such names are exempt from the
relevant laws and regulations and therefore free for general use.

Product Liability: The publisher can give no guarantee for information about drug
dosage and application thereof contained in this book. In every individual case the
respective user must check its accuracy by consulting other pharmaceutical
literature.

Filmset from Disk by Goodfellow & Egan Ltd. Cambridge
Printed by The Alden Press, Osney Mead, Oxford

2128/3916–54321 (Printed on acid-free paper)

Preface

This book is intended as an introduction to the drug treatment of cancer.

It is almost ten years since the last edition was written. In the intervening time, there have been numerous developments in cancer chemotherapy and in order to cover these the majority of the text has been completely revised and rewritten. In addition, two new chapters have been introduced, one on the safe handling of cytotoxic drugs and the other on biological response modifiers. In order to incorporate this new information without any undue increase in the length of the text the chapters on a combined approach to treatment have been omitted. This is not because interdisciplinary collaboration is no longer considered important but is a reflection of the fact that, in most centres, it has become the norm in cancer management and its central role in successful treatment no longer needs to be stressed quite so strongly.

The four chapters in the last edition which dealt with the team approach to cancer therapy have been replaced by a single chapter on the place of chemotherapy in the overall treatment of cancer. Unfortunately, despite all the innovations of the last decade, it has become increasingly clear that much of the promise offered by drug treatment during the 1960s and 1970s has not been fulfilled. Although drugs give excellent results and are mandatory in the cure of certain tumours, these successes have largely been restricted to uncommon cancers. As a result, when looking at potentially curative treatment in numerical terms, chemotherapy still remains very much the junior partner to surgery and radiotherapy. In the last three chapters, therefore, the emphasis is on defining the present role of chemotherapy in the management of individual tumour types, stressing not only its achievements but also indicating the limitations of current treatment.

The relatively limited range of indications for cancer chemotherapy, coupled with the fact that virtually all cytotoxic agents carry potentially lethal toxicities, mean that the use of these drugs should still be restricted to expert clinicians with specific oncological training. For this reason, as in previous editions, relatively few details of drug dosages and treatment regimes in individual diseases have been given.

Many aspects of the drug treatment of cancer remain uncertain or controversial and, in what is intended as a purely introductory text, it is impossible to cover all these areas at great length. Detailed references have been deliberately avoided but a bibliography is provided, listing a selection of recent review articles on individual topics and giving details of books providing a particularly useful overview of certain aspects of the subject, for those who wish to pursue specific items in more depth.

Finally, I would like to thank Gordon Muir-Jones, at Farmitalia Carlo-Erba, for his encouragement to undertake this new edition of my book and his support during its completion.

Birmingham   T. J. Priestman
September 1988

Contents

Section 1 The Principles of Cytotoxic Drug Therapy

Chapter 1 Principles of Tumour Growth

Introduction 3
Mitosis 4
Nucleic Acids 5
Duplication of DNA 7
The Cell Cycle 7
Kinetic Implications of the Cell Cycle 9
Cell Loss 10
Resting Cells 11
Natural History of Tumour Growth 13
Cell Numbers and Tumour Growth 14

Chapter 2 The Effects of Cytotoxic Drugs on Normal Tissues

Introduction 15
Bone Marrow 17
Gastrointestinal Tract 19
    Direct Effects on the Gastrointestinal Epithelium 19
    Nausea and Vomiting 19
The Skin 20
The Unborn Child 21
Male Fertility 22
Female Fertility 23
Carcinogenicity 23

Chapter 3 The Pharmacology of Cytotoxic Drugs

Introduction 27
Drug Dosage 27
Alkylating Agents 28
    Mode of Action 28
    The Nitrogen Mustards 29
    Aziridines 34

Dimethanesulphonates 34
Nitrosoureas 35
Epoxides 35
Antimetabolites 36
Mode of Action 36
The Vinca Alkaloids 41
Mode of Action 41
Antimitotic Antibiotics 42
Anthracycline Antibiotics 42
Non-anthracycline Antibiotics 44
Miscellaneous Compounds 46
Non-classical Alkylating Agents 46
Anthracenediones 49
Epipodophyllotoxins 49
Hydroxyurea (Hydrea) 49
Amsacrine (Amsidine, AMSA) 50
Enzyme Therapy 50

Chapter 4   The Rationale of Cytotoxic Drug Therapy

Introduction 53
Tumour Regression and Cure 53
Single Agent Continuous Therapy 54
Fractional Cell Kill 55
Combination Chemotherapy 56
Intermittent Chemotherapy 57
Scheduling of Therapy 61
Tumour Growth Fraction 62
Drug Access 62
Drug Resistance 62
Timing of Cytotoxic Therapy 62
Adjuvant Therapy 62
Neo-adjuvant Therapy 63
Choice of Drugs for Combination Therapy 64
Cytotoxic Drugs and the Cell Cycle 65
Alternating Non-cross Resistant Regimes 66
Drug Dose 66
Reduced Toxicity 68
Continuous Infusion Chemotherapy 68

Chapter 5   The Management of the Side Effects of Cytotoxic Drugs

Introduction 71
Routine Precautions 71
Bone Marrow Toxicity 72
Leucopenia 72
Thrombocytopenia 73
Anaemia 74

Nausea and Vomiting 74
Alopecia 76
Drug Extravasation 77
Antagonism of Cytotoxic Action 78
  Leucovorin 78
  Mesna 79

Chapter 6   The Safe Handling of Cytotoxic Drugs

Introduction 81
Precautions During the Preparation of Injectable
  Cytotoxic Drugs 82
Precautions for Administration of Cytotoxic Drugs 83

Chapter 7   Resistance to Cytotoxic Drugs

Introduction 89
General Factors 89
  Timing of Drug Administration 89
Anatomical Isolation 90
  Drug Antagonism 91
  Antibody Formation 91
Cellular Factors Causing Drug Resistance 91
  Alterations to the Cell Membrane 92
  Increased Drug Deactivation 92
  Loss of Drug Activation Process 92
  Increased Production of Target Molecule 93
  Change in Enzyme Specificity 93
  Production of Non-essential Competitors 93
  Alternative Biochemical Pathways 93
  Repair of Cytotoxic Damage 94
Prevention of Drug Resistance 94
Cross Resistance 95

**Chapter 8   Alternative Methods of Cytotoxic Drug
Administration**

Introduction 97
Central Venous Access 97
Intra-arterial Therapy 98
  Head and Neck Cancer 99
  Hepatic Metastases 100
  Malignant Melanoma and Soft Tissue Sarcomas 101
  A Note on Terminology 101
Intrapleural Therapy 102
Intraperitoneal Therapy 103
  Control of Ascites 103
  Control of Tumour 103
Intravesical Therapy 104

Intrathecal Therapy 105
Topical Therapy 106

**Chapter 9   The Development and Assessment of New
Cytotoxic Drugs**

Introduction 107
Preclinical Testing 107
Clinical Evaluation 109
    Phase I Studies 109
    Phase II Studies 109
    Phase III Studies 110
Criteria of Assessment 110
    Cure 110
    Survival 111
    Response 113
    Palliation 114
Conclusion 116

Section 2   Biological Response Modifiers

Chapter 10   Biological Response Modifiers

Introduction 121
Monoclonal Antibodies 122
Lymphokines 124
    Interferons 124
    Interleukin-2 125
    Tumour Necrosis Factor 125
Oncogenes 126
Growth Factors 127

Section 3   The Principles of Endocrine Therapy

**Chapter 11   The Development and Rationale of Endocrine
Therapy**

Introduction 131
The Cellular Basis for Hormonal Sensitivity in Breast Cancer   131
Clinical Correlations of Oestrogen Receptor Status 133
Carcinoma of the Prostate 134
Endometrial Carcinoma 134
Renal Cell Carcinoma 135
Carcinoma of the Thyroid Gland 136
Glucocorticoids and Cancer Therapy 136

Chapter 12   The Clinical Pharmacology of Endocrine Drugs

Anti-oestrogens 139
    Tamoxifen 139

Inhibitors of Steroid Synthesis 141
    Aminoglutethimide 141
Oestrogens 142
Androgens 143
Anti-androgens 143
    Cyproterone Acetate (Androcur, Cyprostat) 143
    Flutamide 143
LHRH Analogues 144
The Progestins 144
The Glucocorticoids 146

Section 4   The Clinical Role of Chemotherapy

Chapter 13   The Place of Chemotherapy in Cancer Treatment

Introduction 151
Advantages and Limitations of Available Treatment
    Modalities 151
The Objectives of Cancer Treatment 152

Chapter 14   Childhood Cancer

Introduction 157
Wilms' Tumour 158
Neuroblastoma 159
Central Nervous System (CNS) Tumours 160
Rhabdomyosarcoma 160
Ewing's Sarcoma 161
Retinoblastoma 162

Chapter 15   Haematological Cancers

Introduction 163
Acute Lymphoblastic Leukaemia 163
Acute Myeloid Leukaemia 165
Chronic Myeloid Leukaemia 167
Chronic Lymphoid Leukaemia 168
    B-cell CLL 168
    Hairy-cell leukaemia 169
Hodgkin's Disease 169
Non-Hodgkin's Lymphoma 172
Polycythaemia Vera 175
Multiple Myeloma 176

Chapter 16   Solid Tumours

Lung Cancer 177
    Small Cell Lung Cancer 177
    Non-small Cell Lung Cancer 178

Carcinoma of the Breast 179
  Early Breast Cancer 179
  Advanced Breast Cancer 181
Gastrointestinal Cancer 184
Genitourinary Cancer 185
  Carcinoma of the Prostate 185
  Carcinoma of the Kidney 186
  Carcinoma of the Bladder 187
  Testicular Cancer 188
Gynaecological Cancer 189
  Carcinoma of the Cervix 189
  Carcinoma of the Endometrium 189
  Carcinoma of the Ovary 190
  Choriocarcinoma 191
Head and Neck Cancer 192
Malignant Melanoma 193
Brain Tumours 193
Osteogenic Sarcoma 194
Soft Tissue Sarcomas 195

Bibliography 197

Subject Index 205

The Principles of Cytotoxic Drug Therapy

Principles of Tumour Growth

Introduction

A cancer represents a population of cells within the body which escapes from normal control mechanisms and continues to increase until, unless previously treated, it leads to the death of the host. In healthy adults, however, many normal tissues contain actively multiplying cells, the replication of which is essential for the processes of repair and replacement. A basic knowledge of the growth patterns of both these normal tissues and malignant cell populations is fundamental to an understanding of the drug treatment of cancer.

Animals and man go through two phases in their growth. From birth to maturity the total number of cells in the body increases with a consequent increase in size and weight: this is normal childhood growth. When this growth is complete and the child becomes an adult, the overall size remains reasonably constant, as does the total number of cells, so no growth is apparent. The behaviour of cells within the body varies greatly in different tissues. In the central nervous system and skeletal muscle, for example, the total cell number reaches a maximum at the time of maturity, and during the rest of life the small number of these cells that are constantly wearing out and dying are not replaced so the cell population slowly decreases. In other tissues, cells are continuously lost in huge numbers but are always replaced. In these tissues, growth is continuing as actively as it ever did in the earlier part of life, but this growth is aimed at repair and replacement, keeping the tissue population constant without increasing the total number of cells in the body. Examples of these continuously proliferating tissues include the skin and the lining of the gut, the cells of which are constantly being worn away and must be replaced. Similarly, the bone marrow is continuously replacing the various cellular components of the blood (which have only a limited lifespan) and may be used as an example to show the scale of cell turnover in normal tissue. Red blood cells have a life span of 120 days, the average red cell count is 5 million cells per cubic millimetre and the average blood volume for a man weighing 70 kilogrammes is 5 litres. This means that the bone marrow has to replace some 2,000 million red cells every day. Yet, despite the vastness of this number, the normal physiological controls of cell growth ensure that the replacement is carried out with great accuracy, so that the number of cells lost is precisely balanced by the number of new cells produced. If this were not so, and too few cells were generated, then anaemia would soon develop; conversely, if too many cells were formed then the equally serious condition of polycythaemia would result. Similar control mechanisms exist in all normally multiplying tissues, ensuring a constant total cell number. The nature of some of these controls and the processes by which cells escape from them to form cancers are considered further in Chapter 10.

Once an individual cell, or group of cells, escapes from these normal constraints the resulting uncontrolled replication leads to the formation of a tumour mass. As this increases in size and age, especially in more rapidly dividing tumours, the cells tend to resemble the parent tissue less and less. They become undifferentiated and lose the specific characteristics which initially distinguished them. The growth will invade and destroy surrounding normal tissues and clumps of cancer cells may break off into the lymphatic vessels or the veins and be carried to distant sites, forming secondary growths or metastases. (It is these two properties – invasion of adjacent structures, resulting in tissue destruction, and the ability to produce metastases – that distinguish cancers from benign growths.) Eventually, if left untreated, involvement of vital organs or general debility will lead to death. Throughout this time, the fundamental process is tumour growth resulting from proliferation of cancer cells no longer responsive to the normal control mechanisms regulating the cell population.

The tumour may be controlled by surgical removal, by killing the growing cells with ionising radiation or by chemical means. Surgery and radiotherapy are only successful if the lesion is still localised so that it may either be completely excised or covered by a field of radiation. These local methods of treatment have only limited value once the disease has disseminated, offering symptom control in certain circumstances but having no potential for cure at this late stage. Chemical methods of ablation may be used for both local and metastatic lesions. Such drug treatment involves either endocrine therapy, altering the hormonal environment of certain tumours and thereby slowing their growth, or the administration of cytotoxic drugs. Cytotoxic drugs act against the tumour by interfering with cell division thereby slowing down or reversing the growth of the cancer. To understand their mechanisms of action and the theories underlying their clinical application the processes of cell division and tumour growth must first be described.

Mitosis

Every cell in the body consists of two components: a nucleus and its surrounding cytoplasm. In the nucleus are the chromosomes carrying the genetic material that will ensure the functional integrity of the cell and also dictate its inherited characteristics. Division of the cell nucleus into two

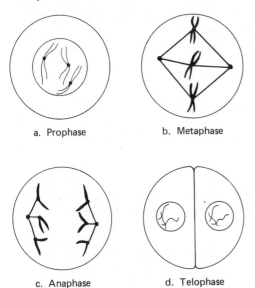

a. Prophase   b. Metaphase

c. Anaphase   d. Telophase   **Figure 1.1.**   The stages of mitosis.

daughter nuclei, therefore, represents the most important event of cell reproduction: it is known as mitosis. The chromosomes only become visible to light microscopy at the time of nuclear division and four stages of mitosis can be recognised (Figure 1.1)

1. Prophase. The chromosomes first become visible as long thin filaments which progressively shorten and thicken. At this stage each chromosome has already split into its two daughter chromosomes or chromatids, each pair being held together by a specialised structure, the centromere.

2. Metaphase. The membrane of the nucleus disappears and an array of microtubules, called the spindle, forms between the opposite poles of the cell. The chromosomes arrange themselves at the middle of the cell by lying across the spindle and are attached to it by the centromeres, forming the equatorial plate.

3. Anaphase. The chromatids separate and move to opposite poles of the spindle.

4. Telophase. The chromosomes elongate and disappear as a new nuclear membrane forms. The spindle also disappears. The cytoplasm then divides.

The period between mitoses, when the cell is apparently at rest, is termed the interphase.

Nucleic Acids

The elucidation of the process of mitosis and the appreciation of the importance of chromosomes as the carriers of genetic material led scientific

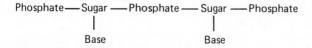

Figure 1.2.   The structure of the DNA chain.

interest to focus on the structure of the chromosomes. It is now known that they are made up of nucleic acids, which are compounds comprising thousands of subunits, termed nucleotides. Each nucleotide comprises three further subunits: a phosphate group, a five carbon (pentose) sugar and a nitrogen-containing base.

There are two forms of a nucleic acid: one has deoxyribose as its sugar unit, is therefore named deoxyribose nucleic acid, or DNA, and is found in the chromosomes; the other has ribose as its sugar, is called ribose nucleic acid, or RNA, and is mainly concerned with protein synthesis within the cell. DNA contains four different nitrogenous bases: the pyrimidines, cytosine and thymine, and the purines, adenine and guanine. RNA also contains four nitrogen bases but thymine is replaced by another pyrimidine – uracil. The nucleotides are arranged in a chain-like pattern (Figure 1.2). The sugar and

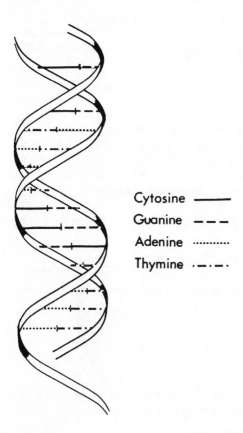

Cytosine ——
Guanine — — —
Adenine ··········
Thymine ·—·—·

Figure 1.3.   The DNA complex.

phosphate groups form alternate links in the chain and the nitrogenous bases are attached to the sugar units, at right angles to the chain.

The DNA complex exists as two such chains which are twisted into a helix and wound round one another in a spiral fashion (Figure 1.3). The two opposing spirals are held together by hydrogen bonds linking the nitrogenous bases, which project into the space between the strands. The nature of the hydrogen bonds joining these base pairs is highly specific. Adenine unites readily with thymine, and guanine with cytosine. The linking of adenine with guanine or cytosine is, however, very difficult and would result in distortion of the helical structure of the DNA macromolecule. Similarly guanine cannot pair with adenine or thymine. Thus, a base on one chain can form hydrogen bonds with one, and only one, of the four possible bases on the other chain. As a result of this phenomenon, if the sequence of bases of one chain is known then those on the other are at once apparent. For example, if a small section of one DNA strand had the base sequence CYT, GUA, THY, THY, AD then the opposite chain must comprise GUA, CYT, AD, AD, THY. This structural configuration is essential for the duplication of DNA.

Duplication of DNA

The sequence of the bases on the DNA chain of the chromosomes carries the genetic code, which determines the structure and function of the cell. At the time of mitosis the nucleus must, therefore, not only double its quantity of DNA but also produce new DNA identical to the old in order to secure genetic continuity.The structure of DNA ensures that this is so and the mechanism of replication is as follows. At various points or replicating sites in the DNA chain the two strands separate by breakage of the hydrogen bonds linking their base pairs. These unpaired bases are then free to pick up other bases from the surrounding medium, but because of the specific nature of the hydrogen bonds, described above, each base can only join with one of the four available. When the bases are paired, linking enzymes bring in the sugar and phosphate groups to complete the new DNA strand which is, therefore, identical to the other parent strand of DNA. Thus each of the initial DNA chains acts as a template for the other, ensuring that the new DNA macromolecule is identical to the old and that there is continuity of structure and consequently transmission of genetic material intact to the next generation (Figure 1.4).

The Cell Cycle

Initially it was thought that the synthesis of DNA was a continuous process throughout the apparent resting, or interphase, period between mitoses. In

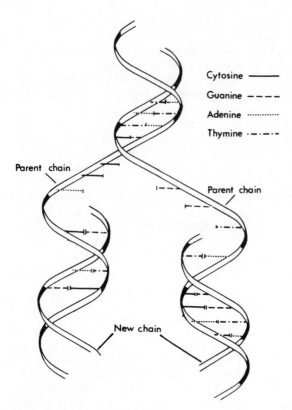

Cytosine ———
Guanine — — — —
Adenine ············
Thymine ·—·—·—·—

Parent chain

Parent chain

New chain

Figure 1.4. The replication of DNA.

the early 1950s it became possible to label the nitrogenous base thymidine with a radioactive marker so allowing its incorporation into the newly formed DNA to be monitored. The results of these experiments showed that DNA synthesis was actually achieved in a relatively short space of time and that, even in rapidly dividing cells, there was a distinct gap during interphase both before and after the period of DNA formation.

This discovery led to the concept of the cell cycle, which is now generally accepted, and comprises the following stages (Figure 1.5):

G_1 – an initial resting phase.

S – the synthetic phase, during which the doubling of the DNA occurs.

G_2 – a second resting phase or premitotic phase.

M – the actual process of mitosis.

In addition, some cells that have the capacity for division may not be actively dividing at the time of observation and are said to be in G_0 phase: they may be considered as temporarily removed from the cell cycle. Suitably stimulated, they would move into the G_1 phase and begin multiplying once again.

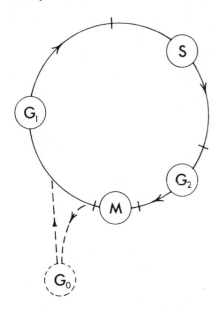

Figure 1.5. The cell cycle.

The use of radioactive thymidine labelling and other techniques that were subsequently developed has led to a vast increase in our knowledge of the events occurring during the cell cycle and of the patterns of growth and proliferation of cells in normal and tumour tissues. The discovery of a discrete phase of DNA synthesis and the subsequent elaboration of the cell cycle have implications both from a therapeutic point of view and also in our general understanding of the way in which tumours grow. This latter aspect has now become a major subject in its own right: the study of tumour kinetics.

Kinetic Implications of the Cell Cycle

The initial studies of cells grown in tissue culture (*in vitro* tests) and investigations of cell growth in living animals (*in vivo* tests) gave similar measurements for the duration of the various phases of the cell cycle. The length of G_1 appeared to be the most variable factor, sometimes being completely absent and, in other cell systems, lasting as long as 30 hours, although most values lay between 5 and 10 hours. S had a more constant time of 6 to 8 hours and G_2 was also reasonably uniform with a duration of 2 to 4 hours. Mitosis was usually completed within 1 hour. Subsequent studies demonstrated that these were minimum values and have suggested that 90 per cent of human tumour cells have cell cycle times (usually abbreviated to T_C) within the range 15 to 120 hours, with an average of 48 hours. It has also been shown that T_C may vary considerably for different cells within the same tumour, thereby giving rise to a kinetic heterogeneity that was not suspected in the earlier experiments.

For many years it was thought that a tumour grew because it consisted of cells which multiplied more rapidly than those in the surrounding normal tissues. If this were so, the T_C of malignant cells should be much shorter than that of replicating normal cells. In fact the average T_C of 48 hours for human tumour cells is, if anything, slightly longer than that of non-malignant cells. So, if the rate of cell division was the only factor determining tumour growth, the cancer would grow at the same rate as, or even more slowly than, normal tissue and would cause no problems. Thus the old idea of a tumour being a mass of very rapidly proliferating cells has been largely abandoned.

This leads to the question of how, then, does a tumour grow? When a normal cell divides, it does so only to replace a cell which has been lost: in this way a constant cell population is maintained. But, as we have already seen, a cancer occurs as a disorder of cell growth in which this particular control mechanism has been lost, so that when a cancer cell divides it adds to the existing number of cells and increases the total population. Thus in a cancer the total cell number is not constant but is continually increasing.

One measure of the rate of tumour growth is the time taken for a given population of malignant cells to double in size. This period is called the doubling time, or T_D. If each passage through the cell cycle results in the formation of two daughter cells then, since we have stated that the T_C for 90 per cent of human tumour cells lies between 15 and 120 hours, the doubling time for the majority of human cancers should be within this range. In fact, observations of the T_C of human tumours have revealed times varying from 96 hours to 500 days. The T_D depends on the histological type of the tumour, its age and whether it is a primary growth or a metastasis. A shorter T_D of under 30 days is usually seen with testicular teratomas, non-Hodgkin's lymphomas and acute leukaemias, whereas common solid tumours, such as squamous cell carcinoma of the bronchus and adenocarcinomas of breast and large bowel, generally have a T_D in excess of 70 days. The T_D for each histological type does, however, vary considerably from patient to patient, although as a general rule metastases have a shorter T_D than their primary tumour and hence grow more rapidly. This may be a genuine observation, indicating the presence of more malignant cell clones in the secondary lesions, or it may reflect the fact that most of these experimental observations are based on lung or skin metastases and these sites may preferentially favour more rapid growth.

These results leave us with a marked discrepancy between T_C and T_D for individual tumours. To explain this difference two other factors affecting tumour growth must be considered: cell loss and resting cells.

Cell Loss

So far, we have assumed that every cell a tumour produces remains within that tumour and continues to produce future generations of cancer cells.

There is now considerable evidence that large numbers of cells produced by a tumour are very rapidly lost from the total population. This cell loss may occur in the following ways:

1. Exfoliation: this is most obvious in tumours of the skin and gastrointestinal tract where friction is continuously wearing cells away from the tumour surface.

2. Hypoxia at the tumour centre: as solid tumours (the carcinomas and sarcomas) increase in size they tend to outgrow their blood supply and the central part of the tumour becomes anoxic, leading to necrosis and cell death.

3. Biologically inadequate cells: tumour growth is abnormal and many of the cells formed are either totally non-viable or else survive but are unable to divide for more than one or two generations.

4. Metastases: tumour cells are capable of amoeboid movements and may infiltrate blood or lymph vessels and be washed away and subsequently form metastases.

5. Host defences: the host's immune mechanisms may destroy variable numbers of tumour cells.The number of cells lost in these ways may represent between 50 and 99 per cent of all those produced by the tumour. The ratio of cells produced to those lost is called the cell loss factor and, for the great majority of cancers, it is between 95 and 99 per cent. This figure looks remarkably high but, considered on the same basis, the cell loss factor for normal dividing tissues is 100 per cent – every cell lost being replaced by one cell only so that zero growth occurs.

A cancer may, therefore, be viewed not as a mass of very rapidly dividing cells but as a tissue replicating at an approximately normal rate which fails to lose a proportion of the cells produced and, therefore, gradually increases in size.

Resting Cells

The normal human bone marrow contains stem cells which are characterised by two properties: the capacity for self-perpetuation through countless cell divisions, and the ability to form committed cells which go on to produce the various blood cell precursors. Despite the vast number of cells which the marrow has to produce it seems that more than 50 per cent of the stem cell population is not actively dividing but resting, in the G_0 phase, out of the cell cycle. These cells have not lost the ability to reproduce and with an appropriate stimulus, such as haemorrhage, the resting stem cells will be recruited into the cell cycle and play an active role in blood cell replacement. It is now clear that a similar situation exists in other dividing cell systems including tumours, where not all cells capable of cell division are actively proliferating. This has led to the concept of the tumour growth fraction, which is the ratio between the number of cycling cells and the total number of cells in the tumour.

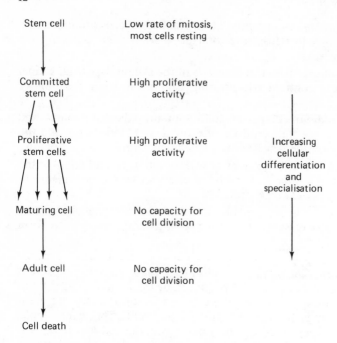

Figure 1.6.   The process of replacement of normal cells.

Measurement of the growth fraction is not easy in human cancers and is liable to a number of errors; however, the figures available at present are as low as 10 per cent, or less, for some sarcomas and carcinomas, increasing to 90 per cent in certain leukaemias and lymphomas.

This concept of a tumour composed of dividing cells and resting cells needs to be taken one step further to give a complete picture. Within the tumour there are the tumour stem cells, or clonogenic tumour cells, which are able to produce an infinite number of future generations of similar cells. These stem cells may either be resting or proliferating. There is another population of replicating tumour cells which are capable only of four or five further divisions because they are limited by some biological flaw: these have been termed "doomed cells". Finally there are those cells which, although they are

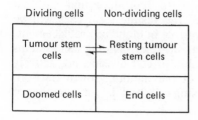

Figure 1.7.   A simple kinetic diagram of a tumour.

alive in the sense that cellular functions are maintained, have no capacity for replication: these are called "end cells".

Thus a tumour is made up of two compartments: dividing cells and non-dividing cells. The dividing compartment comprises stem cells and doomed cells. The non-dividing compartment comprises resting stem cells and end cells (Figure 1.7).

Clearly a tumour with a large dividing cell component has a high growth fraction and is likely to increase in size more rapidly than a tumour with few dividing cells and a low growth fraction.

Natural History of Tumour Growth

Tumour growth depends on three factors: the cell cycle time, the growth fraction and the cell loss factor. The resultant of these three is the tumour doubling time. We can now ask whether the doubling time is a constant for any given tumour; in other words does a tumour grow at the same rate throughout its life?

Experiments where tumour cells are grown in tissue culture have shown that the doubling time remains constant and in a given period of time the percentage increase in tumour size is the same. This means a tumour that doubles its size in two days will have quadrupled in four days and be eight times its original volume in six days.This pattern of proportional increase in size with unit time is termed exponential growth. It is seen in some human leukaemias but not in solid tumours, where it appears that the rate of growth slows as the tumour increases in size and age. In general the larger the tumour the longer its doubling time. This progressive decrease in the rate of growth is common to a number of biological systems and is often referred to as Gompertzian growth, after Benjamin Gompertz, the English mathematician who first described the process in 1825.

The full explanation for the slowing of growth is still uncertain, but tumour blood supply is certainly an important factor. As the cancer increases in size many cells will be pushed further away from the capillaries and become relatively anoxic. Experiments have shown that, although cell cycle times are not affected by oxygen depletion, the growth fraction is reduced by 50 per cent or more under anoxic conditions. Thus there is probably a kinetic micro-architecture within tumours, with those regions nearest to blood vessels multiplying more rapidly than those at a distance from capillaries. As the tumour grows the latter inevitably predominate with a consequent slowing in the doubling time.

Shrinkage of a cancer, by either chemotherapy or irradiation, would be expected to reduce the extent of anoxic areas and might, therefore, result in an increase in the growth rate of residual cells. There is some evidence that this is the case and that reduction of a tumour cell population by treatment reduces the doubling time with a return to the more rapid growth seer in the earlier stages of its development.

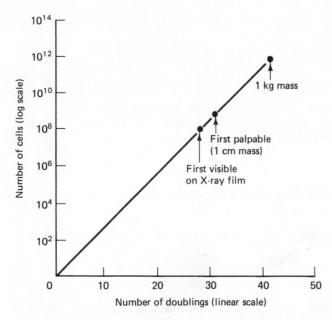

Figure 1.8.   Tumour cell population in relation to clinical detectability.

Cell Numbers and Tumour Growth

One of the main difficulties of measuring human tumours *in vivo* is that such growth only becomes large enough to observe at a late stage in their life. The human body contains about 5×10^{13} cells. A cancer is usually assumed to originate from a single aberrant cell, but it will not become clinically detectable until there are at least 10^9 tumour cells, with a mass of about 1 gramme (although most cancers are far larger than this by the time they are diagnosed). The patient usually dies before the tumour reaches 10^{12} cells (Figure 1.8).

In any patient, therefore, the growth of a cancer is only detectable and observable during the last 10 to 14 of its 35 to 40 doubling times. Although there have been some attempts to project backwards from these observations to determine the early events in the life history of tumours, even if we allow for the rate of change of growth with age, what actually occurs during the major part of a cancer's lifespan is the subject of theory and speculation.

Recent developments in molecular biology and genetics have given some insight into the possible events in the very earliest stages of tumour development. These discoveries could have far-reaching implications for the drug treatment of cancer and are reviewed in Chapter 10.

Chapter 2

The Effects of Cytotoxic Drugs on Normal Tissues

Introduction

We have defined a tumour as a population of dividing cells in which the number of cells produced exceeds the number of cells lost. Cytotoxic drugs act by interfering, in a variety of ways, with cell division. As a result of this inhibition the production of new cells is reduced, with a reversal in the ratio of cells produced to cells lost. As a consequence the total cell population progressively diminishes and the cancer regresses. Once this process is established one would hope to go on giving cytotoxic drugs for a sufficient length of time to destroy all the cells in a tumour and cure the patient. In practice, with a few exceptions, this is not possible. Two factors prevent the universal success of chemotherapy in cancer treatment: drug resistance (see Chapter 7) and the dose-limiting toxicity of cytotoxic drugs.

All cytotoxic drugs share two properties: an ability to inhibit the process of cell division and an inability to distinguish between normal and malignant cells. This means that when a cytotoxic drug is introduced into the body it will attack not only dividing cancer cells but also normal cells which are proliferating as part of the physiological processes of repair and replacement. If given indiscriminately cytotoxic drugs would destroy entire populations of normal cells with fatal results. The clinical application of these agents is, therefore, an exercise in differential poisoning – the object being to kill the cancer before one kills the host!

In addition to their shared activity against replicating tissues, individual cytotoxic agents have their own specific toxicities. These may often be severe, or even potentially lethal, and they include cardiac damage, pulmonary infiltration, neurotoxicity, liver impairment and renal failure. These toxicities are summarised in Table 2.1 and are considered in more detail in relation to individual agents in Chapter Three. The remainder of this chapter considers the general effects of cytotoxic action on proliferating tissues.

The rate of normal cell proliferation varies considerably in different tissues (Table 2.2). Some tissues virtually cease replication once the body reaches maturity whilst others produce millions of new cells every day up to the time

Table 2.1.   Summary of short and medium-term toxicities of cytotoxic drugs

	Myelosuppression	Gastrointestinal toxicity	Neurotoxicity	Alopecia	Pneumonitis and/or lung fibrosis	Cardiotoxicity	Renal damage	Hepatotoxicity	Skin changes	Endocrine abnormalities	Haemorrhagic cystitis	Acute allergic reactions
Nitrogen mustard	3	2	1	1					1			
Cyclophosphamide	2	2		2	1	1		1	1	1	2	
Ifosfamide	2	2	2	2	1			1			3	
Melphalan	3	2		1	1				1			
Chlorambucil	2	1		1	1			1				
Thiotepa	2	1										
Hexamethylmelamine	2	2	2									
Busulphan	2				2				1	1		
Nitrosoureas	3	2		1	1			1	1			
Methotrexate	2	2	2	1	1		1	1	1			
5-Fluorouracil	2	2	1	1	1				1			
Cytosine arabinoside	2	2	1				1	1				1
6-Mercaptopurine	2	1						2				1
6-Thioguanine	2	1						1				
Vincristine	1	2	3	1						1		
Vinblastine	2	1	1	1					1			
Vindesine	2	1	2	1					1			
Doxorubicin	3	2		3		3			1			
Daunorubicin	3	2		2		3						
Epirubicin	2	1		2		2						
Actinomycin-D	2	2							1			
Mitomycin-C	2	2			1		1					
Bleomycin		1		2	3				1			1
Cisplatinum	2	3	2				3					1
Carboplatin	3	2	1				2	1				1
Mitozantrone	2	1		1		1		1				
Dacarbazine	1	2	1	1				1	1			1
Procarbazine	2	2	1					1				
Etoposide	3	2		2								1
Asparaginase	2	2	2	1	1			2	2		2	1
Amsacrine	3	2	1	1		1		1				
Hydroxyurea	2	1							1			

1. Occasional or minor side effect.
2. Common or moderately severe side effect.
3. Invariable or dose limiting side effect.

of death. The effects of cytotoxic drugs will be most obvious in those normal tissues which are dividing most rapidly, and it is the appearance of toxicity to these tissues which limits the usefulness of the drugs at the present time. Such toxicity is usually seen acutely in the days or weeks during and immediately after treatment, but long-term damage also occurs and two areas of increasing importance are the late effects of cytotoxics on children who undergo chemotherapy and the carcinogenic potential of some agents.

Table 2.2. Examples of normal tissues with differing proliferative properties

Tissues which are continuously rapidly proliferating	Bone marrow Gastrointestinal mucosa Hair follicles Testicular germ cells
Tissues which are continuously slowly proliferating	Tracheobronchial epithelium Vascular endothelium
Tissues which proliferate in a cyclical fashion	Glandular female breast cells Endometrial lining of uterus
Tissues with the capacity to proliferate after injury	Liver Bone
Non-proliferating tissues	Skeletal muscle Cardiac muscle Cartilage Neurones

Bone Marrow

Normal human tissues in which there is continuous cellular repair and replacement comprise two cell populations: the stem cell and the differentiated cells.

Stem cells are capable of producing many generations of similar cells. It was originally thought that their reproductive capacity was infinite, but it is now clear that after some 25 to 40 doublings stem cells lose the ability to divide. Therefore, in order to maintain the processes of repair and replacement only a few clones of stem cells are dividing at any one time: when these become exhausted, other clones move from a resting to a mitotic phase to take their place.

The differentiated cells arise from the progeny of the stem cells and undergo a number of chemical and physical changes which result in a loss of their power of reproduction and in the development of those specialised characteristics which enable them to play a specific role in the body.

This system is clearly demonstrated by the bone marrow. The stem cell population is continually producing cells which will mature and differentiate into red blood cells (erythrocytes), certain types of white blood corpuscles (granulocytes or polymorphonuclear leucocytes) or platelets. The stem cell from which an erythrocyte develops is indistinguishable from those producing granulocytes or platelets but the mature erythrocyte is a highly specialised cell completely different in appearance, structure and function from granulocytes and platelets.

These mature cells, however, have no ability to reproduce and once fully differentiated have only a limited life span. Cytotoxic drugs inhibit cell division but have little or no effect on mature differentiated cells. Therefore when a cytotoxic drug is given, the red cells, granulocytes and platelets in the circulation at that time are unaffected. It is the stem cell population which is attacked and as a result the number of new cells produced is diminished.

The stem cells in the bone marrow are dividing extremely rapidly and measurements indicate that they have a doubling time of only 15 to 24 hours (compared with anything from 4 to 500 days for cancers). The bone marrow is, therefore, extremely sensitive to cytotoxic drugs and almost any agent given in sufficient quantities will affect a large number of dividing cells at a sensitive stage of the cell cycle and deplete the bone marrow stem cell population. The effect of this depletion is seen clinically in a fall in the numbers of the various cells circulating in the blood.

Erythrocytes have a life span of some 120 days, the platelets 9 to 10 days and the granulocytes probably only survive for 4 to 5 days. If no new cells were produced then the granulocyte population would be reduced to zero within a week. Similarly the platelets would have disappeared within a fortnight but the erythrocytes would not vanish completely for 4 to 5 months. Thus the first effect which is seen in the peripheral blood after a cytotoxic drug is given is a fall in the white cell count, usually occurring between 3 to 7 days after treatment. If a sufficiently large dose has been administered then in some 7 to 14 days a fall in the platelet count will occur. A fall in the red cell count would not be detectable for some 6 to 8 weeks and is rarely seen after a single dose of a cytotoxic drug. The reason for this is that, provided the dose was not excessive, bone marrow recovery will take place within a week or so after drug administration and the stem cell population will have returned to normal before any significant fall in the peripheral red cells is apparent. If, however, the dose of drug was so excessive as to cause complete bone marrow failure then the patient would die from infection (due to lack of granulocytes) or haemorrhage (due to lack of platelets) long before anaemia developed.

In some instances, if the drugs are given in a low dose but administered continuously, so that there is little opportunity for stem cell recovery, signs of bone marrow suppression may be delayed for many months. When they do appear, however, all three cell populations, erythrocytes, granulocytes and platelets, become diminished at approximately the same time and the clinical picture is that of total marrow failure or aplastic anaemia, which may or may not be reversible if the drug is stopped.

Not all cytotoxic drugs affect the bone marrow to the same degree or at the same time. Some drugs almost invariably produce marrow suppression at therapeutic doses (melphalan, doxorubicin, mitozantrone) whilst at least one agent (bleomycin) has no reported bone marrow toxicity. Similarly some drugs cause very rapid falls in the white cell count, apparent within two or three days of treatment (nitrogen mustard), whilst with others this toxicity may not be apparent for three or four weeks after the drug is given (CCNU and carboplatin). This spectrum of toxicity applies to all the possible effects of cytotoxic drugs on proliferating tissues the likelihood and severity of side effects varying greatly with individual agents.

Gastrointestinal Tract

Direct Effects on the Gastrointestinal Epithelium

The cells lining the gastrointestinal tract are continually being worn away by the passage of food and have constantly to be replaced from a stem cell population. The rate of division of stem cells in the gastrointestinal tract is only slightly lower than that of the bone marrow cells and so these tissues are also extremely sensitive to the action of cytotoxic drugs. The symptoms caused by the drugs will vary at different parts of the gastrointestinal tract. Nausea and vomiting is a major toxicity with many agents but the mechanism underlying chemotherapy-induced emesis is complex and probably only partly due to the direct action of drugs on the gastrointestinal tissues: it is considered in more detail below. Oesophagitis, diffuse ileitis, colitis and proctitis may all occur, but oral mucositis is the commonest manifestation of gastrointestinal toxicity after nausea and vomiting.

The buccal mucosa is replaced every 4 to 7 days and is subjected to considerable local trauma in an environment rich in pathogenic bacteria. These factors predispose to the development of oral mucositis some 3 to 4 days after cytotoxic administration. Initial symptoms include pain, tingling, dryness of the mouth and loss of taste. These then progress to frank ulceration which may affect the lips, tongue, palate and gums. This reaches a peak at about 7 days and then gradually subsides unless infection or haemorrhage supervenes. The frequency and severity of mucositis is related to the dose of the drug and the schedule of administration: it is most commonly seen with methotrexate, 5-fluorouracil, cytosine arabinoside, actinomycin-D, bleomycin and doxorubicin.

Nausea and Vomiting

The causes of chemotherapy-induced emesis are still not fully understood but it is recognised that at least three factors are involved:

1. The action of cytotoxic drugs on the replicating cells in the lining of the gastrointestinal tract, particularly those located in the small intestine, results in stimulation of the vagus nerve and release of various gastrointestinal hormones. These include 5-hydroxytryptamine (serotonin) which stimulates specific receptors ($5HT_3$ receptors) in the upper small intestine which, in turn, lead to stimulation of the vagus nerve.

2. Cytotoxics directly stimulate receptors in the chemoreceptor trigger zone, which is located in the floor of the fourth ventricle in the brain.

3. There is an input from higher cerebral centres. This is most clearly demonstrated by the development of anticipatory nausea and vomiting, where patients who have already experienced emesis following cytotoxic administration develop further nausea and vomiting shortly *before* subsequent courses of treatment are given.

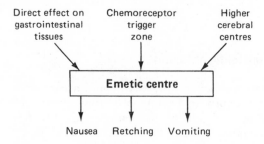

Figure 2.1.   The mechanism of cytotoxic drug-induced emesis.

These various stimuli cause the release of a number of neurotransmitters, including methionine, catecholamines, prostaglandins, dopamine and enkephalin. These then act on the emetic centre, which is situated in the area postrema of the brain stem. Efferent pathways from the emetic centre then mediate the three separate but interrelated components of emesis: nausea, retching and vomiting. These pathways are summarised in Figure 2.1.

The risk of nausea and vomiting varies with different cytotoxics and usually increases with increasing doses of the drug. Emesis usually occurs from 2 to 8 hours after drug administration but the duration and severity of symptoms depends not only on the cytotoxic(s) given and their dose but also varies considerably from patient to patient. Drugs which almost invariably cause considerable nausea and vomiting at therapeutic doses include cisplatinum, nitrogen mustard, dacarbazine, ifosfamide and doxorubicin, whereas agents such as bleomycin, the vinca alkaloids and anti-metabolites are only mildly emetic.

The Skin

Contact with the external environment leads to erosion of the superficial layers of the skin, which have to be continuously replaced. Also some 60 to 90 per cent of the hair follicles are actively dividing at any one time, with doubling times of approximately 24 hours. As a result alopecia, due to suppression of the cells in the hair follicles, is often seen during cytotoxic therapy. Hair loss usually becomes apparent some three to five weeks after starting treatment. The process is reversible and the hair will regrow after treatment although this may take some three to five months and the texture and colour of the hair may be altered. Occasionally hair follicles become resistant to cytotoxic treatment and hair growth will reappear whilst the patient is still on treatment. Again there is a spectrum of activity between different cytotoxics: some agents very rarely cause alopecia (cisplatinum, mitomycin-C and chlorambucil, for example) whereas others almost inevitably lead to complete alopecia (doxorubicin, etoposide, ifosfamide).

Although a number of cytotoxic agents carry the risk of specific skin toxicities (see Chapter 3), generalised skin reactions are uncommon with chemotherapy but a number of drugs will cause severe local reactions if they leak into cutaneous tissues during intravenous administration. Such extravasation causes stinging and burning at the site of injection which, depending on the drug and the extent of the leakage, may progress to severe local inflammation with tissue necrosis and ulceration. This is often very slow to heal and may even require skin grafting. Vesicant cytotoxics are listed in Table 6.1 and the management of extravasation is considered in Chapter Five.

The Unborn Child

The development of the unborn child goes through two phases. From about ten days after fertilisation until the end of the eighth week of pregnancy is the period during which the various organs in the body are formed. Damage to the embryo during this period will lead to gross deformity (a teratogenic effect) which may prove fatal. By the end of the eighth week organogenesis is complete and the remainder of pregnancy is a period of foetal growth. The possible complications of cytotoxic therapy will therefore depend upon the stage of pregnancy at which treatment is given. Drug administration during the first eight weeks could lead to deformity or abortion; treatment after that time might cause inhibition of growth and prematurity.

Many experimental studies have been undertaken in a variety of animals to test for the teratogenic effects of cytotoxic agents and most of the drugs in general use have been shown to have such an effect. The relevance of these findings to humans is uncertain and very few reports are available on the outcome of cytotoxic administration to pregnant women: generalisations from such limited data are unreliable. Methotrexate, however, has consistently demonstrated a teratogenic effect and has actually been used as a means of inducing abortion. It should never be given during the first three months of pregnancy. Cyclophosphamide, chlorambucil and busulphan have all been reported to have a teratogenic effect in humans but normal offspring have also been recorded following treatment throughout pregnancy with these agents. Although teratogenic in other animals, the vinca alkaloids have not been shown to cause damage to the human embryo in the few patients treated.

The administration of cytotoxic drugs during the latter part of pregnancy, when organogenesis is complete, appears to be less hazardous. The drugs will cross the placenta and the foetus will experience similar toxic effects to the mother, but at low doses no long-term damage is apparent in the great majority of cases, although premature labour and infants underweight at birth are common.

A further theoretical hazard of cytotoxic administration during pregnancy is the risk of genetic damage with the production of chromosomal defects which may lead to complications in later life or future generations. Only long-term follow-up over several generations will quantify this risk but the few projected assessments made have suggested that the risk to the individual is slight and the effect on the genetic load of the population as a whole is negligible. With the expanding use of cytotoxic therapy and the increasing number of long-term survivors it is possible that this balance may change but it is too early for these very delayed effects of treatment to be apparent.

In summary, the safest advice is that cytotoxic therapy should be avoided completely during the first three months of pregnancy. After the first trimester the risk of severe damage from treatment is considerably reduced but use of these agents inevitably involves some risk.

Male Fertility

In adults the testis performs two separate functions: the epithelium of the seminiferous tubules produces spermatozoa while the interstitial cells of Leydig have an endocrine role, synthesising and secreting the male hormone testosterone. The germinal epithelium of the seminiferous tubules is replicating continuously throughout adult life and is therefore highly susceptible to the antimitotic effects of cytotoxic drugs. Following administration of these agents there is depletion, or even aplasia, of the germinal epithelium, with marked reduction in the number of spermatozoa, often progressing to their complete disappearance (azoospermia). Clinically these effects appear as a noticeable decrease in the volume of the testis (the seminiferous tubules make up about 75% of the normal testis) and infertility. The activity of the Leydig cells, however, is little altered and testosterone production is not noticeably affected so there are no changes in secondary sexual characteristics.

The precise effects of individual agents on male fertility have only been studied in detail with respect to a number of alkylating agents, such as cyclophosphamide and chlorambucil, and specific drug combinations, particularly those used in Hodgkin's disease. The likelihood of testicular damage with other drugs, although very probable, is less well defined. From the studies that are available it is clear that the risk of sterility is related to the cumulative dose of the drug given. For example, azoospermia appears universal when the total dose of chlorambucil exceeds 400mg and that of cyclophosphamide 6 to 10 grammes, when the drugs are given as single agents. Giving alkylating agents in combination with other cytotoxics almost certainly results in azoospermia at far lower cumulative doses.

The recovery of spermatogenesis following chemotherapy is unpredictable. As a general rule the greater the dose of drug given the smaller the chance of regaining fertility. Even in those patients who do recover it may be several years following their treatment before spermatogenesis is restored and the duration of this recovery period appears, once again, to be dose-related. Given the unpredictability of cytotoxic action on male fertility it is an essential precaution that all young men about to undergo chemotherapy are given the opportunity of sperm banking prior to starting treatment.

Female Fertility

Like the testis, the mature ovary also has a dual role: the release of ova and the production of the hormones oestrogen and progesterone. In contrast to the spermatozoa, however, the female ova are all formed during intrauterine life rather than being continuously produced throughout adulthood. Each ovum becomes covered by two layers of specialised cells – the theca and granulosa cells, which are responsible for oestrogen synthesis – to form the primordial follicles. At the time of birth each ovary will contain 150,000 to 500,000 such follicles. From the menarche to the menopause the first half of each menstrual cycle will consist of follicular growth and maturation, with increasing oestrogen secretion, culminating in the release of a single follicle at ovulation. Thereafter the follicle lodges in the uterus to form the corpus luteum, which secretes increasing levels of progesterone as well as some oestrogen, until the end of the cycle.

Cytotoxic therapy causes ovarian fibrosis with destruction of the follicles, resulting in amenorrhoea and sterility. These changes also result in a fall in oestrogen levels and menopausal symptoms, such as hot flushes, may occur together with other features of oestrogen deficiency such as atrophy of the vaginal epithelium. The effects of single agent chemotherapy on ovarian function are, once again, best documented for alkylating agents and it is clear that the incidence of problems is directly related to dose. With combination therapy including alkylating agents, approximately 50% of women develop amenorrhoea, although the figure varies with different regimes. Age is a very important factor in determining both the susceptibility to amenorrhoea and the likely restoration of ovarian function after treatment. For patients under the age of 40 years far higher doses are tolerated before ovarian function is affected and the likelihood of normal periods returning after treatment is far greater than for older women.

Carcinogenicity

Clear evidence for the development of second cancers in man following cytotoxic therapy has now emerged from observations on two groups of patients: the long-term survivors of certain cancers (Hodgkin's disease, some childhood malignancies and ovarian carcinoma) who received cytotoxics as part of their treatment and patients with non-malignant conditions who received prolonged immunosuppressive therapy involving the administration of cytotoxics (some transplant patients and a number of patients with severe rheumatoid arthritis and related conditions).

It is still impossible to quantify precisely the risk of second malignancy after chemotherapy, nor do we know all the factors which contribute to that risk. This is partly because we are still dealing with a relatively small patient population on whom very prolonged follow-up observations are necessary in order to gain a complete picture. Furthermore, virtually all the data so far available come from retrospective surveys which are inherently incomplete and relatively inaccurate. Nevertheless, a number of interim conclusions may be drawn:

1. The risk of second cancer formation varies with different drugs. At present cytotoxics may be grouped in three categories: firstly, those that have clearly been shown to be carcinogenic in *clinical* studies (these include nitrogen mustard, cyclophosphamide, chlorambucil, melphalan, the nitrosoureas, procarbazine and thiotepa); secondly, agents which have demonstrated some carcinogenicity in *laboratory* tests but not, as yet, in *clinical* series (these include bleomycin, doxorubicin, actinomycin-D, cisplatinum and the vinca alkaloids); finally, a number of drugs which have, so far, shown no evidence of carcinogenicity in either the laboratory or in patients (these include methotrexate, 5-fluorouracil and cytosine arabinoside).

2. Dose and scheduling may well affect the likelihood of second cancer formation. There is some evidence that the greater the dose the greater the risk. There are also indications that the same total dose is more carcinogenic if given as a constant small dose over a long period of time rather than as a few intermittent high-dose treatments.

3. There is very clear evidence that combining cytotoxics and irradiation leads to a greater chance of second tumour formation than with either modality used alone. There is also limited evidence that combinations of potentially carcinogenic cytotoxics carry an increased risk compared to single agent therapy.

4. There is a latent interval between the administration of chemotherapy and the appearance of second cancers. Leukaemias occur at an average of six years after therapy but are uncommon at ten years or more after treatment. Lymphomas occur a little later and solid tumours a little later still. It is impossible to give average times of onset for the lymphomas and solid tumours because a number of long-term studies suggest that their incidence is still rising some 15 years after initial treatment so that the latent interval between cytotoxic administration and the appearance of these tumours may be twenty years or even longer.

5. Precisely quantifying the chances of second cancer development is virtually impossible at the present time but figures from two large series do give an indication of the risks involved. One study, carried out by the National Cancer Institute in the USA, looked at 5,455 women who had received adjuvant therapy with alkylating agents following a diagnosis of ovarian carcinoma and compared them with a control population. The women treated with cytotoxics were found to have a significantly higher risk of developing acute leukaemia. Although the statistical evidence for that risk was quite unequivocal the actual number of cases was relatively small; 15 women actually developed acute leukaemia in the treated group as compared to an expected incidence of 1.62 cases. In a second series following the progress of 907 patients with Hodgkin's disease over a fifteen year period 56 second cancers were seen (including leukaemias, lymphomas and a spectrum of solid tumours) compared to the 9.5 that would have been expected in a normal

population. Although the absolute number of second cancers is greater than in the ovarian series many of these patients also had radiotherapy, compounding the carcinogenic hazard, and *all* would have died from their Hodgkin's disease had treatment not been given. Furthermore many of the second cancers which did develop could be successfully treated with appropriate therapy.

Two explanations which are unrelated to treatment with either radiotherapy or cytotoxics may be offered for an increased incidence of second tumours: certain cancer patients may have a genetic susceptibility to tumour formation, or the appearance of a second malignancy may be part of the natural history of the original disease. The concept of genetic susceptibility has been extensively studied in survivors of childhood cancer and it does seem that this is a factor in the development of second primary tumours, but even when allowance is made for this it is still clear that there is an increased incidence of second cancers that is attributable to treatment. The fact that virtually all paediatric tumours involve the use of combined modality therapy with both irradiation and chemotherapy makes it almost impossible to apportion relative carcinogenic risks to these two types of treatment. The place of genetic susceptibility in the aetiology of second tumours in adults is still uncertain. In the past it has been suggested that in certain conditions, such as the lymphomas, the appearance of leukaemia after apparently successful primary treatment may simply represent an extension of the natural history of the disease – that there is some underlying malignant process in the marrow or lymphoid system which, at first, manifests itself as myeloma or lymphoma but after the initial treatment subsequently reappears as a leukaemia. Studies, which admittedly are retrospective, in both myeloma and lymphoma have now shown that prior to the introduction of cytotoxic treatment and radiotherapy the incidence of leukaemia in these diseases was no different to that seen in control populations. Although it is possible that the increased survival time resulting from the introduction of these therapies has modified the natural history of the disease, the fact that treatment has increased the risk of second cancers is inescapable.

The mechanism for carcinogenesis by antitumour drugs is still a subject of intensive research, but two main theories have evolved. The first relates to a direct action of certain drugs on cellular DNA. The suggestion is that agents which attack, or bind intimately with DNA in the cell nucleus, may not always kill that cell but might cause sublethal damage which, in the long-term, will result in abnormal cell division and hence cancer formation. Support for this concept comes from the observation that cancer formation, following chemotherapy, in animals and man has been seen mainly with those agents which react directly with DNA – (the alkylating agents and certain antimitotic antibiotics) – whereas agents which have no direct effect on DNA, such as methotrexate and 5-fluorouracil, have not shown any carcinogenic potential. In addition, there are a number of structural similarities between some metabolites of alkylating agents and cytotoxic antibiotics and recognised chemical carcinogens which are known to cause cancer by direct attack on the structure of DNA. In contrast purine antimetabolites, which do not react with DNA, have been associated with the development of tumours in patients

receiving these drugs as immunosuppressive therapy following transplantation. This introduces the second explanation for cytotoxic carcinogenicity – immunosuppression. It has been suggested that the body is constantly
producing small cancers which are recognised by the immune system and
destroyed by host defences at a very early stage in their development: this is
the theory of immune surveillance. If this theory is correct then prolonged
immunosuppression would inhibit host defences and allow such tumours to
grow unchecked. Because of their action on the bone marrow, and in
particular on the white cells, all cytotoxics cause some degree of immunosuppression and could enhance tumour development in this way.

To summarise a complex and still incompletely understood subject one may
say that there is unequivocal evidence that cytotoxic therapy with certain
drugs, particularly alkylating agents, increases the risk of second cancers. In
terms of the absolute numbers of second cancers seen, however, the risk is
relatively small. If chemotherapy is essential for cure or to prolong survival in
those with incurable disease then the risk of second cancers should not restrict
its use. It is in the field of adjuvant therapy, where many long-term survivors
will be seen and the benefits of cytotoxic therapy are still often uncertain, that
the greatest caution needs to be exercised in deciding whether to use these
drugs.

Chapter 3

The Pharmacology of Cytotoxic Drugs

Introduction

After the first promising results of cytotoxic treatment during the 1940s there was a tremendous surge of activity to discover new anticancer agents in the hope of finding the ideal drug that would eradicate the tumour whilst having no harmful effects on normal tissue. Forty years later this hope has yet to be fulfilled, but the search for new cytotoxics has yielded many thousands of compounds with possible therapeutic applications. Somewhat less than forty of these are in common use today.

These agents may be classified as follows:

1. Alkylating agents
2. Antimetabolites
3. Vinca alkaloids
4. Antimitotic antibiotics
5. Miscellaneous compounds

This classification is primarily biochemical and it has been generally assumed that drugs in the same class have similar mechanisms of action against dividing cells. The appearance of cross-resistance between drugs in different groups and the realisation that some compounds have several different modes of action have made the distinction between classes less clearcut than was originally supposed. Nevertheless the classification forms a convenient basis for discussing cytotoxic drugs and is still generally accepted.

Drug Dosage

For the majority of cytotoxic agents it is impossible to quote a fixed dose suitable for every patient as the amount of drug given may vary greatly in different diseases and different treatment protocols. The timing of drug administration is a further variable; an agent may be given three times daily in one condition and once every six weeks in another. The drug doses quoted in this chapter are intended only as an indication of the dose range employed in the commoner treatment regimens. Details of the preparation and administration of intravenous infusions of cytotoxics are given in Chapter 6.

Initially, drug doses were given simply in grammes or milligrammes but, in an attempt to tailor schedules more specifically to meet the needs of individual patients, they are now more frequently given in terms of body weight (mg per kg) or body surface area (mg per m^2). This latter method is considered the most accurate, and special tables, called nomograms, are available which will give the patient's surface area from measurements of their height and weight.

Alkylating Agents

Mode of Action

In the First World War mustard gas (sulphur mustard) was a weapon in trench warfare. It was noted at the time that, in addition to the very damaging caustic effects of the gas, a number of casualties developed a profound fall in their white cell count with damage to marrow and lymphatic tissue. With the end of hostilities medical interest in sulphur mustard waned and the possible therapeutic implications of these observations was overlooked. It was not until the Second World War, when military interest led to further studies on toxic gases, that a possible clinical application for sulphur mustard was suggested. In leukaemia and the lymphomas the underlying pathological process is excessive white cell formation by either the bone marrow or the lymphatic system. A group of clinicians in the USA argued that if sulphur mustard destroyed these tissues in healthy subjects then it might do the same for those suffering from cancer. In 1946 the first studies of cytotoxic therapy for lymphoma were reported in the USA. The initial results were encouraging. The agent used was nitrogen mustard, closely related to the original sulphur mustard but less irritant to normal tissue. These initial favourable results were the first steps on the path of the development of cytotoxic chemotherapy.

Nitrogen mustard is an alkylating agent. Within twenty years of its first therapeutic application over three thousand other alkylating agents were identified for evaluation in cancer treatment. Of these three thousand, fewer than a dozen are in common use today.

An alkyl group is the chemical structure that results when an aliphatic hydrocarbon loses one of its hydrogen atoms. The simplest of all alkyl groups has the formula CH_3. An alkylating agent is a compound that contains an alkyl group and is able to use that group to combine with other molecules by covalent bonds. At its simplest the general formula for an alkylating reaction, or alkylation, may be expressed as follows:

$$R-CH_2-X + Y = R-CH_2-Y + X$$

Biologically active alkylating agents are those capable of alkylating at body temperature and pH. The alkylating agents used in cancer therapy form covalent bonds with a number of biologically active molecules including nucleic acids, proteins, amino acids and nucleotides and have the potential to damage cell membranes, deplete amino acid stores and inactivate enzymes. It has been shown that these drugs attack both a number of enzymes taking part in protein synthesis and also the linking enzymes which are needed for the construction of new DNA strands on their parent templates. Alkylation prevents these enzymes from carrying out their biological role within the cell and so stops the formation of new DNA which, in turn, inhibits mitosis. It is generally considered, however, that a more important action of these drugs in arresting cell division, is the formation of cross-linkages between DNA chains.

One of the sites most susceptible to attack by the therapeutic alkylating agents is the nitrogen atom at the N-7 position on the purine base guanine. The most effective drugs in cancer treatment possess not one but two alkyl groups and are termed bifunctional alkylating agents. The molecular distance between the two alkyl groups is such that they can each bind to a guanine base on the two separate strands of the DNA chain where a turn in the helix brings them close together. In this way the alkylating agents form bridges, or cross-linkages, between opposite guanine bases, binding the DNA strands together and preventing them from separating at the time of DNA replication. In addition, at those points in the DNA chain where separation does occur, alkylating agents will attach to any free guanine bases and prevent them from acting as templates for the formation of new DNA. By these means DNA replication and subsequent cell division are inhibited.

The therapeutic alkylating agents come from five different chemical families: the nitrogen mustards, aziridines, dimethanesulphonates, nitrosoureas and epoxides.

The Nitrogen Mustards

Nitrogen Mustard (Mustine Hydrochloride)

Nitrogen mustard was the first cytotoxic to be used clinically and its formula is shown in Figure 3.1. The two arms bearing the potentially active alkyl radicals are linked by a nitrogen atom to which is attached a methyl group, CH_3. The other nitrogen mustards differ from the parent compound by having alternative chemical groups substituted for the methyl group. Nitrogen mustard has a half-life in the plasma of only a few minutes and has an extremely rapid action. Its clinical usefulness is limited by its severe toxicity. Bone marrow suppression and nausea are almost inevitable after even the smallest thera-

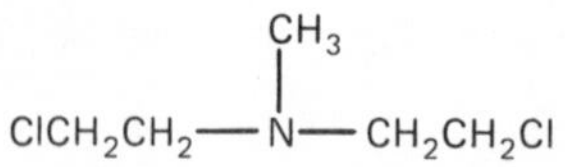

$$CH_3$$
$$ClCH_2CH_2 \!-\!\!\!- N \!-\!\!\!- CH_2CH_2Cl$$

Figure 3.1. Structural formula of nitrogen mustard.

peutic doses. The drug is also extremely corrosive and following intravenous injection the vein should be flushed through with saline to ensure adequate distribution. If the drug escapes from the vein local cellulitis, which is extremely painful, occurs and soft tissue necrosis may develop. If the same vein is used for repeated injections then thrombosis of that vein is likely.

Lymphoid tissue is particularly susceptible to nitrogen mustard and its present day use is virtually confined to the treatment of Hodgkin's disease and some other lymphomas. Because of its very rapid action it is occasionally used in clinical emergencies such as superior vena cava obstruction by carcinoma of the bronchus. Average doses are 5-6mg/m^2.

Cyclophosphamide (Endoxana)

The rationale for the development of this drug was the observation that tumour tissue contains relatively high concentrations of phosphoramidases compared to normal tissue. Therefore, if an alkylating agent could be produced that remained inert until activated by these enzymes it would exert its effect principally at the tumour site, where activation takes place, and have little effect on normal tissue. In theory cyclophosphamide was such an agent, requiring oxidation and other enzyme-mediated transformations for conversion to a number of metabolites with alkylating activity. In practice, it was found that tumour cells *in vitro* could not activate the drug and that an initial conversion by microsomal enzymes in the liver was required. Although details of the resulting metabolites were unclear, these early findings cast doubt on the original rationale for the drug's development.

Modern techniques have now defined the metabolism of cyclophosphamide more clearly (Figure 3.2). Enzymatic hydroxylation in the liver results in the formation of 4-hydroxycyclophosphamide: this spontaneously converts to aldophosphamide and the two molecules form an equilibrium. Non-enzymatic cleavage of aldophosphamide produces acrolein and phosphoramide mustard. Aldophosphamide also undergoes enzymatic conversion to carboxyphosphamide. Phosphoramide mustard, 4-hydroxycyclophosphamide and aldophosphamide are all cytotoxic, but current results suggest that it is phosphoramide mustard which accounts for the clinical activity of cyclophosphamide. Carboxyphosphamide is the major urinary metabolite but phosphoramide mustard, aldophosphamide, 4-hydroxycyclophosphamide and acrolein are also found in the urine.

Cyclophosphamide has proved one of the most valuable cytotoxic drugs and, at one time or another, has been used in the treatment of almost every kind of cancer, frequently with considerable success. Diseases in which it is of particular value include carcinoma of the breast and carcinoma of the bronchus.

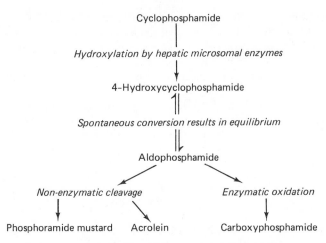

Figure 3.2. Summary of the metabolism of cyclophosphamide.

Bone marrow suppression and gastrointestinal toxicity are seen with cyclophosphamide therapy but are less severe than with nitrogen mustard. In particular it has been noted that cyclophosphamide selectively spares the megakaryocytes (which form the platelets) and thus carries a reduced risk of thrombocytopenia. Cyclophosphamide will also cause alopecia, the risk increasing with higher doses of the drug. As with other cytotoxics the hair will grow again following completion of treatment.

One toxicity unique to cyclophosphamide and its close relative ifosfamide is haemorrhagic cystitis. This varies in severity from mild cystitis to severe bladder damage with massive haemorrhage. The toxicity is due to excretion in the urine of metabolites which have a direct irritant effect on the bladder mucosa and it is thought that acrolein and 4-hydroxycyclophosphamide are the most harmful of these metabolites. The risk of haemorrhagic cystitis is increased by poor hydration and it is important to ensure that those patients receiving cyclophosphamide have a good fluid intake and high urine output. Dose is another factor and when this exceeds $1g/m^2$ mesna should be given simultaneously (see Chapter 5). Prolonged therapy may lead to insidious fibrosis of the bladder wall, though this frequently causes no symptoms. There have also been claims that long-term therapy may lead to bladder cancer but this suggestion remains controversial.

Cardiac damage is another complication when high doses of the drug are used. Patients receiving 100–200mg/kg of cyclophosphamide over 48 hours or less have shown complications ranging from minor ECG changes to acute intractable cardiac failure. Acute fluid retention, probably due to damage to the renal tubules, may also occur with high doses, particularly in children. This is usually a self-limiting and reversible phenomenon which responds to diuretics. Other uncommon side effects which have been reported with this drug include liver toxicity, skin and nail pigmentation, diarrhoea, dizziness, thyroid dysfunction and the syndrome of inappropriate secretion of anti-diuretic hormone.

Cyclophosphamide may be given orally or intravenously. The process of hepatic activation is quite rapid with peak alkylating activity appearing 2 to 3 hours after intravenous administration. The presence of liver secondaries may delay the achievement of this peak level, but the drug remains in the circulation until metabolised so the overall effectiveness of a given dose will not be reduced.

The dose of cyclophosphamide varies greatly. Long-term oral administration may employ doses as low as 50mg daily whilst in some acute situations as much as $2g/m^2$ may be given by intravenous infusion over 24 hours.

Ifosfamide (Mitoxana)

Ifosfamide is structurally similar to cyclophosphamide, the only difference being a change in position of a chloroethyl group (Figure 3.3). The metabolism and mechanism of action of the two agents is similar. Ifosfamide mustard is probably the active metabolite, equivalent to phosphoramide mustard (see above). The spectrum of clinical activity for ifosfamide is still being defined, but it has shown promising results in cervical and endometrial cancer, soft tissue sarcomas, bronchogenic carcinoma and testicular teratomas.

Initially urotoxicity, with haemorrhagic cystitis, was the dose-limiting toxicity of ifosfamide but the introduction of mesna (see Chapter 5) has meant that this complication may now be avoided. Bone marrow suppression is marked,

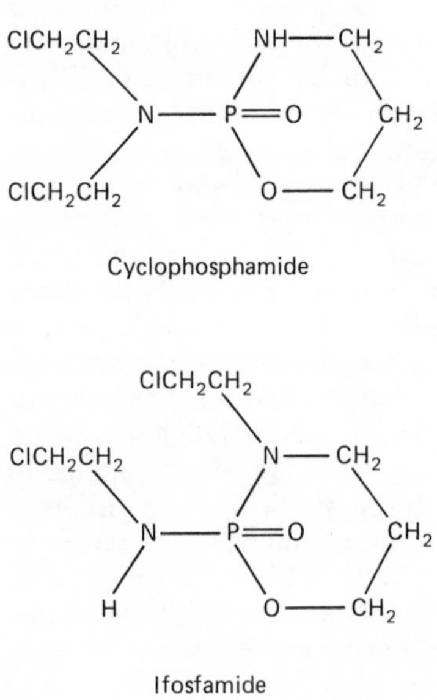

Cyclophosphamide

Ifosfamide

Figure 3.3. Structural formulae of cyclophosphamide and ifosfamide.

with no evidence of platelet sparing. Alopecia occurs in most patients. The severity of nausea and vomiting is dose related and can be very intense at high doses. Neurotoxicity with an encephalopathy, characterised by somnolence, disorientation, confusion, lethargy and occasionally fatal coma, may occur and is more likely in patients with poor hydration, inadequate renal function and low serum albumin levels. With careful patient selection this complication may usually be avoided (see Chapter 5). Cardiotoxicity has not been reported. Dose schedules have varied considerably but most regimes give the drug by intravenous infusion at 1.5–2.5g/m^2 per day for 3–5 days.

Melphalan (Phenylalanine Mustard, Alkeran, L-PAM)

This drug was first produced in Great Britain and the USSR in 1953. Structurally, melphalan has the nitrogen mustard molecule with the essential amino acid phenylalanine replacing the methyl group. It was hoped that the presence of an essential amino acid would lead to the drug being selectively concentrated in dividing cells, where large quantities of amino acids are required for protein synthesis prior to mitosis. In practice, however, there is no evidence that the presence of phenylalanine alters the distribution of the drug.

Melphalan is less widely used than cyclophosphamide but has proved of value in the management of multiple myeloma and carcinoma of the ovary. It has also been used for limb perfusion in the treatment of soft tissue sarcomas (see Chapter 8). Bone marrow suppression is its most marked toxic effect but nausea, vomiting and alopecia also occur with larger doses. The drug may be given orally at a dose of 2–10mg daily or by intravenous injection, the commonest regime being 1mg/kg given every four to six weeks.

Chlorambucil (Leukeran)

This drug was also first synthesised in Great Britain in 1953. Animal experiments revealed that it was particularly active against lymphoid tissue and appeared not only to destroy proliferating cells but to attack mature circulating lymphocytes. This action helps to account for its considerable clinical value in the treatment of chronic lymphatic leukaemia and lymphomas. It has been less widely used for solid tumours although it is of value in ovarian carcinoma.

Nausea and vomiting are uncommon at the usual dose levels and bone marrow toxicity is the dose-limiting side effect. A number of patients given low doses of the drug for several years have developed irreversible bone marrow failure leading to fatal aplastic anaemia. Alopecia, dermatitis, pulmonary fibrosis and liver damage are uncommon complications. The drug is given orally with daily doses ranging from 2 to 10mg.

Aziridines

Thiotepa (Triethylene Thiophosphoramide)

Thiotepa is the only member of this group of alkylating agents in general clinical use. It is a derivative of triethylene melamine which is an alkylating agent originally used in the textile industry, where its property of forming cross linkages between adjacent macromolecules led to increased fibre strength. Although various successes have been claimed for the drug it is now little used apart from instillation into body cavities to control malignant pleural effusions or ascites, or into the bladder in patients with extensive superficial bladder cancer. It is partially absorbed from these sites and does have a myelosuppressive effect. It is, however, more soluble and less damaging to the marrow than many other alkylating agents and so is particularly suitable for intracavitary use. The standard dose for intracavitary administration is 30 to 60mg.

Hexamethylmelamine

This drug, which is a structural analogue of triethylene melamine, is not marketed in Great Britain but has shown some promise in clinical trials for ovarian carcinoma, breast and lung cancer. One interesting observation is that it does not appear to be cross-resistant with other alkylating agents; this has led to speculation that it may have additional modes of action other than alkylation, possibly as an antifolate. Nausea and vomiting are the dose limiting side effects but marrow suppression also occurs, as does neurotoxicity which may take the form of either lethargy and depression, or peripheral neuropathy.

Dimethanesulphonates

Busulphan (Myleran, Myeleran)

Busulphan is the only member of this group of alkylating agents to remain in general clinical use. Its value lies in apparent selective action against granulocytes and its main clinical use is in the management of chronic myeloid (granulocytic) leukaemia. It is also useful in the treatment of polycythaemia vera, thrombocythaemia and some cases of myelofibrosis.

Bone marrow suppression is the principal toxic action but there are very important, less common side effects. Patients on treatment for many months may develop pulmonary fibrosis. This process may be reversed if regular chest radiographs are taken and the fibrosis noted at an early stage, at which point the drug can be stopped and steroid therapy instituted. If it is not recognised, and the treatment is continued, progressive irreversible fibrosis will result in severe respiratory insufficiency, which may prove fatal. Skin pigmentation may also occur with the deposition of melanin, especially on exposed areas, pressure areas, skin creases, the axillae and the nipples. This is a similar distribution to that seen in Addison's disease (adrenal gland insufficiency) and adrenal failure has been reported as a rare complication of busulphan therapy. Another very rare complication is cataract formation. The drug is given orally, usually at a dose of 2 to 4 mg daily.

Nitrosoureas

The nitrosoureas are a family of cytotoxic agents originating from the National Cancer Institute's drug development programme in the USA. The three most important members of the family are BCNU (bischloroethylnitrosourea, Carmustine), CCNU (cyclohexylchloroethylnitrosourea, Lomustine) and methyl-CCNU (methylcyclohexylchloroethylnitrosourea). These drugs have alkylating activity which is thought to be their major cytotoxic action. In addition their metabolites are able to inhibit the enzyme DNA polymerase and prevent the repair of DNA strand breaks and RNA synthesis.

These agents are lipid soluble and pass the blood brain barrier. They have, therefore, been used, with some success, in the management of cerebral tumours. They have also been extensively evaluated in the treatment of gastrointestinal adenocarcinoma, lung cancer and lymphoma but it is only in the latter condition that they have found a regular place in treatment protocols. One of the disadvantages of these drugs which makes them difficult to use in combination regimes is dose-related delayed bone marrow toxicity, with leucopenia and thrombocytopenia often not becoming fully apparent until 4 to 6 weeks after dosing. The other major side effect is gastrointestinal disturbance with nausea and vomiting. Renal and hepatic damage have also been reported as has pulmonary fibrosis.

One other nitrosourea which, like methyl-CCNU, is not generally available in the UK, is streptozotocin. This compound is of interest as it has a specific toxicity to beta cells in the pancreas and shows a significant clinical activity against islet cell carcinomas of the pancreas. The dose limiting toxicities of this drug are gastrointestinal disturbance and nephrotoxicity; bone marrow suppression is less marked than with other nitrosoureas.

BCNU is given by intravenous infusion at a dose of 200mg/m^2 every 6 weeks and CCNU is given orally at a dose of 100–150mg/m^2 every 6 to 8 weeks.

Epoxides

These are a group of alkylating agents chemically similar to the aziridines. No members of this group are generally available in Great Britain at present but two compounds, dianhydrogalactitol and dibromodulcitol, have shown some antitumour activity in preliminary clinical trials.

Antimetabolites

Mode of Action

The antimetabolites were the second family of cytotoxic drugs to be discovered and the first clinical results were reported by Sidney Farber and his colleagues in the USA in 1948. The general principle of their anticancer action is as follows.

Before a cell can divide it must build up large reserves of nucleic acid and protein. For this synthesis to take place various essential metabolites must be present in the cell to form the subunits from which the larger molecules will be built. The antimetabolites are compounds with a very similar chemical structure to certain of these essential metabolites and are either incorporated into new nuclear material in their place, or combine with vital enzymes in an irreversible fashion, thereby inhibiting any further biological activity. As a result of this substitution either the new nuclear material will be unable to fulfil its function or enzyme inhibition will prevent protein synthesis. This breakdown in synthesis or functional integrity of essential molecules will prevent cell division. Many antimetabolites have been produced and studied but only five are in general use today.

Methotrexate

Methotrexate is a folic acid antagonist and is closely related to aminopterin, the drug that Farber used in 1948 (Figure 3.4). A number of tetrahydrofolates are essential co-factors in the synthesis of both purines and pyrimidines. These co-factors are formed by the enzymatic reduction of folic acid. An essential stage in this process is the reduction of dihydrofolic acid to tetrahydrofolic acid. This reduction is carried out by the enzyme dihydrofolate reductase (Figure 3.5). Methotrexate is structurally very similar to folic acid and, furthermore, has an affinity for dihydrofolate reductase 100,000 times greater than folic acid. Thus if a cell contains methotrexate, the enzyme will take it up in preference to folic acid. The methotrexate-dihydrofolate reductase complex that results is almost inseparable, so once it is formed the enzyme is inactivated. If dihydrofolate reductase is inactivated, tetrahydrofolates cannot be synthesised and purine and pyrimidine formation is arrested.

Methotrexate was first employed in the treatment of acute leukaemia, with good results, and is still used in the management of this disease. The greatest success has been in choriocarcinoma where giving methotrexate, as a single agent, has resulted in cure in a high percentage of women. It has also been of value in many solid tumours and is said to be particularly active against squamous cell carcinomas.

The principal side effects of methotrexate are myelosuppression and gastrointestinal disturbance. The latter takes the form of mucositis rather than nausea and vomiting. Usually the earliest manifestation of toxicity is oral

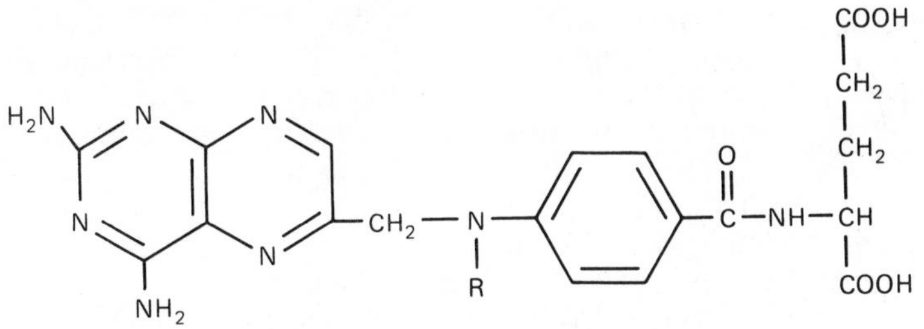

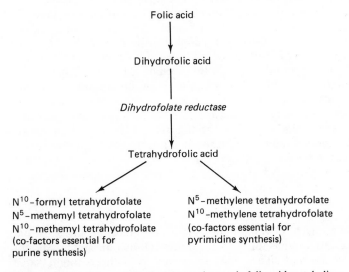

Methotrexate (R$=$CH$_3$)
Aminoterin (R$=$H)

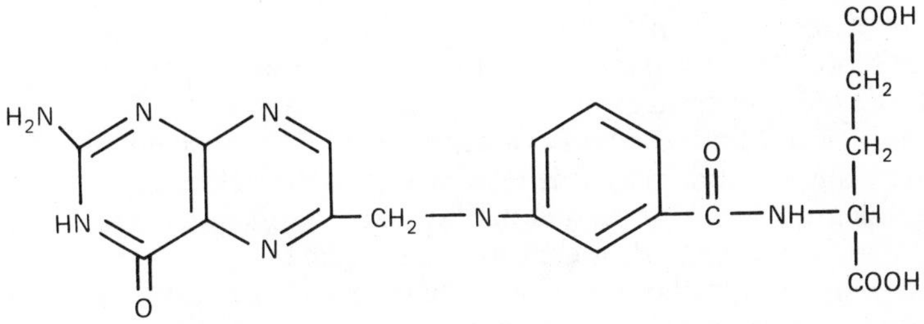

Folic acid

Figure 3.4. The structural similarity of methotrexate, aminopterin and folic acid.

Folic acid

↓

Dihydrofolic acid

|

Dihydrofolate reductase

↓

Tetrahydrofolic acid

N^{10}-formyl tetrahydrofolate
N^5-methemyl tetrahydrofolate
N^{10}-methemyl tetrahydrofolate
(co-factors essential for
purine synthesis)

N^5-methylene tetrahydrofolate
N^{10}-methylene tetrahydrofolate
(co-factors essential for
pyrimidine synthesis)

Figure 3.5. The place of dihydrofolate reductase in folic acid metabolism.

soreness frequently progressing to ulceration of the buccal mucosa. The small intestine is also particularly susceptible to methotrexate and occasionally severe complications such as haemorrhage and perforation occur. Liver damage, occasionally resulting in cirrhosis, has been reported and appears to be more common with long term oral therapy. Renal damage may also occur. This is more frequent with intermittent high-dose regimes where precipitation of methotrexate in the kidney has been noted. A non-specific, self-limiting, pneumonitis has also been described as an occasional side effect.

It is possible to reduce the incidence of serious side effects from methotrexate therapy by giving folinic acid after treatment (see Chapter 5). The drug is only partially metabolised and is largely excreted, unchanged, in the urine. For this reason patients with poor renal function, in whom excretion will be delayed, are at risk of developing severe, if not fatal, toxicity and it is essential to exclude gross renal impairment before giving methotrexate. Methotrexate is also taken up by, and slowly released from, ascitic and pleural fluid. As a result patients with gross pleural effusion or ascites will maintain higher blood levels of the drug for longer times than normal and are at greater risk of side effects. Despite all routine precautions methotrexate toxicity may still occur and is almost always related to delayed plasma clearance of the drug. For this reason it recommended that when high doses are given serial measurements of plasma methotrexate levels are carried out so that toxicity may be anticipated and appropriate action taken.

Methotrexate is given intrathecally in some leukaemias and lymphomas to treat, or prevent, central nervous system involvement. A variety of side effects have been described following such therapy. These include an acute chemical arachnoiditis (headache, nuchal rigidity, vomiting and fever), a subacute syndrome occuring after 2 to 3 weeks (motor paralysis of the extremities, cranial nerve palsies, seizures or coma), and a chronic demyelinating encephalopathy (with limb spasticity, dementia and, in severe cases, coma). The cause of these toxicities is unknown and they are not reversed or arrested by folinic acid.

Methotrexate may be given orally, intravenously or intrathecally. The dose varies from 2.5mg daily, by mouth, in some long-term maintenance regimes to as much as 5g by intravenous infusion, followed by folinic acid. A number of laboratory studies have shown interactions between methotrexate and other cytotoxics; these have not, as yet, been demonstrated to have any clinical significance but may be summarised as follows: methotrexate enhances 5-fluorouracil and cytosine arabinoside activation, vincristine enhances methotrexate uptake but 5-fluorouracil given prior to methotrexate inhibits its antifolate activity.

5-Fluorouracil

5-Fluorouracil was a logical development from an observation, in 1954, that chemically-induced hepatomas in the rat utilised uracil in much greater quantities than did normal liver. This suggested that there might be a biochemical difference between the normal and malignant cells and hence a possible target for antimetabolite therapy. 5-Fluorouracil was the first of a series of fluoropyrimidines made with this objective. It remains the most important of these compounds and is also the simplest, consisting of a uracil molecule with a fluorine atom substituted for the number five hydrogen atom. This minimal alteration in chemical structure allows it to inhibit cell division in two ways. Firstly, it blocks the enzyme thymidilate synthetase, which converts deoxyuridilic acid to thymidilic acid. This is an essential step in pyrimidine synthesis and 5-fluorouracil therefore prevents the formation of thymine and cytosine, thereby arresting the production of new DNA. Secondly, normal RNA contains uracil, in place of thymine. Because of its close structural similarity 5-fluorouracil is incorporated into RNA in place of uracil and as a consequence inhibits RNA synthesis. At present it is not clear which of these two effects is the more important in 5-fluorouracil's anticancer activity.

5-Fluorouracil has been used mainly in the management of solid tumours and, in particular, the adenocarcinomas of the gastrointestinal tract and breast. The principal toxic effects are bone marrow suppression and sickness, both of which may be severe if high doses are given. Uncommon side effects include alopecia, skin rashes, cerebellar ataxia, conjunctivitis and chest pain.

Absorption following oral administration is erratic and 5-fluorouracil is usually given intravenously. When used as a single agent the most effective schedule has proved to be an initial 5-day loading course followed by single weekly doses. Originally the loading course was given as daily bolus injections of 10–15mg/kg but it has subsequently been found that higher doses, of 20–30mg/kg day, may be administered by continuous intravenous infusion over the 5-day period with less toxicity than the lower dose bolus regime.

Cytosine Arabinoside (Cytarabine, Cytosar)

Cytosine arabinoside is an analogue of the nucleoside deoxycitidine and has a number of effects on DNA formation. It inactivates the enzyme DNA polymerase, which is responsible for binding thymine to the DNA strand during DNA synthesis and thereby inhibits both DNA formation and repair. Cytosine arabinoside is also directly incorporated into the DNA chain with the result that the DNA is more susceptible to degradation and its replication is prevented.

Cytosine arabinoside is strongly myelosuppressive and this is its main toxic effect. Nausea, vomiting, diarrhoea and oral ulceration frequently occur during drug administration but subside rapidly thereafter. Reversible hepatic dysfunction, with elevation of liver enzymes and mild jaundice, may also be seen.

Clinical use of the drug is confined mainly to leukaemia and it is particularly valuable in acute myeloid leukaemia in adults. It is given by intravenous injection or infusion in doses of 100mg/m^2 during remission induction. The schedule of administration is critical to the success of therapy with continuous infusions or bolus doses every 8 hours being superior to once-daily injections.

6-Mercaptopurine (Purinethol)

6-Mercaptopurine is a purine antagonist and was developed by Hitchings and Elion in the USA in the early 1950s. The drug undergoes enzymatic transformation to its active form, thioinosinic acid. Thioinosinic acid then goes on to inhibit a number of different enzymes which catalyse the early stages of purine synthesis and thus prevents the formation of adenine and guanine.

6-Mercaptopurine is used mainly in the treatment of leukaemia, particularly acute lymphatic leukaemia. The commonest side effect is marrow suppression. Hepatotoxicity has been seen in a number of patients, both cellular liver damage and biliary stasis having been reported. The drug is metabolised in the liver and excreted in the urine. The enzyme xanthine oxidase plays a vital role in the degradation of 6-mercaptopurine and this enzyme is inhibited by the drug allopurinol. In some cancers, especially leukaemia and the lymphomas, there may be a very rapid breakdown of tumour tissue with cytotoxic treatment, resulting in high uric acid levels. As this secondary hyperuricaemia may lead to renal failure, patients who might develop this complication are given allopurinol since this drug lowers the serum uric acid level. It is important to realise that patients who receive allopurinol concurrently with 6-mercaptopurine will have delayed metabolism of the latter agent. In this situation the dose of 6-mercaptopurine should be reduced by 70 per cent to avoid the risk of excessive toxicity. The drug is given orally and typical doses in maintenance therapy are 50–100mg daily.

6-Thioguanine (Lanvis)

6-Thioguanine is another purine antagonist and was also developed by Hitchings and Elion. Like 6-mercaptopurine it requires enzymatic conversion to its active form, 6-thioguanylic acid, which inhibits a number of enzymes involved in purine synthesis. There is evidence for a number of other potentially cytotoxic actions of this drug, including direct incorporation into DNA, inhibition of glycoprotein synthesis and inhibition of messenger-RNA formation.

6-Thioguanine is used principally in the treatment of myeloid leukaemias. Its major toxicity is bone marrow suppression. Gastrointestinal disturbance and hepatic dysfunction are also seen but less commonly than with 6-mercaptopurine. Unlike 6-mercaptopurine concurrent allopurinol therapy does not enhance 6-thioguanine toxicity as xanthine oxidase is not required for its inactivation. 6-Thioguanine is given orally and a typical dose is 2–2.5mg/kg daily.

The Vinca Alkaloids

Mode of Action

Alkaloids are nitrogenous bases which are formed in plants and many of them have medicinal properties: cocaine, morphine, quinine and atropine are all plant alkaloids. The vinca alkaloids are derived from the periwinkle plant, *Vinca rosea*, and three of these, vincristine, vinblastine and vindesine, have anticancer activity. All three drugs have a similar mechanism of action, the fundamental element of which is binding to tubulin. Tubulin is an intracellular protein that polymerises to form microtubules. Microtubules are involved in a number of functions including mitosis, transport of solutes, cell movement and maintaining the structural integrity of the cell. In mitosis the microtubules form the cell spindle on which the chromatid pairs are arranged during metaphase. Vinca alkaloid binding prevents the polymerisation of tubulin and microtubule formation. This means that spindle formation is inhibited and mitosis is halted at metaphase (hence the alternative name for these drugs: metaphase arresting agents). Although this probably represents the principal cytotoxic action of the vinca alkaloids they have also been shown to have a number of other properties which might be relevant including inhibition of thymidine incorporation into DNA and uridine incorporation into RNA.

Vincristine (Oncovin)

Vincristine has proved particularly valuable in the management of leukaemias and lymphomas and has been incorporated into combined drug regimes for a number of solid tumours, most notably in breast cancer. One reason for its use in combination therapy is its relative lack of myelosuppression. At low doses (less than $1mg/m^2$) the drug actually has a stimulating effect on megakaryocytes and may result in an increase in circulating platelets.

The most important side effect of vincristine is neurotoxicity. This most frequently presents as a peripheral neuropathy which may be either sensory, motor or mixed. Initially symptoms and signs are slight – tingling and numbness in the fingers and toes or loss of deep reflexes (the ankle jerk is usually the first to disappear). If these are ignored and treatment continued, irreversible neuropathy may occur with footdrop, wristdrop and other more severe paralyses. It is, therefore, essential that patients receiving vincristine are questioned about sensory disturbance and have their reflexes tested prior to each injection. Constipation, which may occasionally progress to paralytic ileus, is a further complication and is thought to be due to autonomic neuropathy. Convulsions, visual disturbances and coma are rare manifestations of vincristine neurotoxicity. Other complications are uncommon but include alopecia and inappropriate secretion of anti-diuretic hormone, resulting in a salt losing syndrome causing weakness and drowsiness.

Vincristine is given by intravenous injection, the usual dose being 1–1.4mg/m^2.

Vinblastine (Velbe)

Vinblastine has been of most value in the management of Hodgkin's disease. It is markedly more myelosuppressive than vincristine and this is its dose limiting toxicity. It is also a very corrosive drug causing a painful cellulitis if it escapes from the vein during administration. Mucositis is another relatively common side effect. Alopecia may occur but neurotoxicity, similar to that of vincristine, is rare and only seen following high doses of the drug. Vinblastine is given by intravenous injection at a dose of about 6mg/m^2.

Vindesine (Eldisine)

Vindesine is the most recently introduced of the vinca alkaloids and has been most widely used in the treatment of malignant melanoma. The main side effects of vindesine are a moderate leucopenia, without thrombocytopenia, and mild neurotoxicity. The latter is primarily sensory. Alopecia has also been reported. The current dose schedule is 3mg/m^2 once weekly by intravenous injection.

Antimitotic Antibiotics

Antibiotics are beneficial in the treatment of infections because they inhibit the multiplication of bacteria. In the search for new antibiotics during the 1940s and 1950s it became apparent that some of the compounds isolated had a similar inhibitory effect on dividing tumour cells and numerous antibiotics with anticancer activity have now been isolated and a number are in common use today. The anthracyclines probably form the most important group but a number of other antibiotics are also of value in cancer treatment.

Anthracycline Antibiotics

Daunorubicin (Rubidomycin, Cerubidin), Doxorubicin (Adriamycin), Epirubicin (Pharmorubicin)

The anthracycline glycosides are pigmented antibiotics produced by different strains of *Streptomyces*. In 1963 the first anti-tumour anthracycline, daunorubicin (Rubidomycin, Cerubidin) was isolated. This drug showed marked activity against leukaemias and stimulated the search for similar compounds with a broader spectrum of anticancer activity. In 1969 doxorubicin (Adriamycin) was isolated and subsequently proved to be one of the most effective of all cytotoxic drugs with activity against a wide range of solid tumours including carcinoma of the breast, bronchogenic carcinoma, gastric cancers and soft tissue sarcomas. Both daunorubicin and doxorubicin have quite marked side effects and a number of analogues have been developed with the object of retaining antitumour activity whilst reducing toxicity. The first of these to become widely available in Great Britain is epirubicin (Pharmorubicin).

The mode of action of the anthracyclines is still not completely understood but at least five potentially cytotoxic effects of these agents have been identified:

1. Intercalation: this means that the molecular structure of the drug is such that it can insert itself between opposing DNA strands, rather like a key fitting into a lock, and bind to specific components of the DNA. This results in disturbance of various DNA functions and, in the case of the anthracyclines, it seems to be mainly DNA and RNA synthesis that are inhibited.

2. Membrane binding: anthracyclines have been shown to bind to various components of cell membranes, leading to altered membrane fluidity and changes in permeability to various ions.

3. Free radical formation: free radicals are compounds that possess an unpaired electron and they are often highly reactive towards DNA and other biologically important macromolecules. Anthracyclines undergo enzymatic transformations which release free radicals within the cell and these can cause breaks in the DNA chain, thereby preventing mitosis.

4. Metal ion chelation: anthracyclines have the ability to chelate, or bind, various metals including copper, zinc and iron. Some of the resulting chelates are thought to be cytotoxic.

5. Alkylation: it has been shown that some metabolites of the anthracyclines act as alkylating agents.

This summary demonstrates the multiple possibilities for cytotoxic activity that the anthracyclines possess, though the relative importance of these various properties in relation to their antitumour effect is still unclear.

Daunorubicin and doxorubicin can cause severe bone marrow suppression and considerable nausea and vomiting. Alopecia is almost universal. A further important side effect of both drugs is cardiotoxicity. This may appear in an acute or chronic form. The acute changes include the appearance of arrhythmias and conduction abnormalities, within a few hours of drug administration, and the "pericarditis–myocarditis syndrome" (tachycardia, cardiac failure and pericarditis) which develops a few days later. The chronic toxicity takes the form of a cardiomyopathy which may result in irreversible, and ultimately fatal, cardiac failure. The development of cardiomyopathy is related to the cumulative dose of the drug and with a total dose of doxorubicin in excess of 550mg/m^2 the incidence of overt cardiac failure approaches 10 per cent. Patients over 70 years of age, those with previous cardiac disease or hypertension and those who have had previous irradiation of the myocardium are at increased risk of cardiotoxicity. Prior to therapy with daunorubicin or doxorubicin all patients should have a clinical examination and an ECG to exclude myocardial disease but the value of serial ECGs during treatment, to monitor toxicity, is doubtful. Although various strategies have been suggested for reducing the risk of cardiac toxicity the only certain way of minimising clinically overt cardiac complications is dose limitation. It has been recommended for daunorubicin that the total dose should be less than 20mg/kg and for doxorubicin the cumulative dose should not exceed 550mg/m².

Epirubicin shares the same pattern of toxicity as daunorubicin and doxorubicin but has been shown to cause much less severe gastrointestinal disturbance at equivalent doses and also to be significantly less cardiotoxic. Its range of clinical activity is still being determined but initial results indicate that it is very similar to doxorubicin.

Non-anthracycline Antibiotics

Actinomycin-D (Cosmogen, Lyovac, Dactinomycin)

In 1940 the actinomycins were identified as bactericidal products of a soil fungus, *Actinomyces*. Actinomycin-D was the most cytotoxic member of the actinomycins and was the first antimitotic antibiotic to be introduced, in 1954. Actinomycin-D appears to act primarily by intercalating with DNA and binding to guanine. The principal result of this intercalation seems to be inhibition of RNA synthesis by the DNA chain which, in turn, prevents protein synthesis and the formation of new DNA.

Actinomycin-D is of value in the treatment of certain paediatric tumours, choriocarcinoma, soft tissue sarcoma and testicular teratomas. Myelosuppression is the dose limiting side effect. Gastrointestinal disturbance with nausea, vomiting, diarrhoea and mucosal ulceration of the mouth and small bowel may all occur. Alopecia is common and acneiform skin eruptions are also seen. Actinomycin-D is a radiation sensitiser and increases the toxicity of radiotherapy when the two treatments are given concurrently. The drug may also provoke radiation recall phenomena, causing inflammatory reactions in previously irradiated areas. The mechanism of radiosensitisation and radiation recall is unkown.

Actinomycin-D is given by intravenous injection and is highly irritant if it escapes from the vein. A typical course comprises 10 to 15 micro-grammes per kg given daily for 4 days and repeated every 3 to 4 weeks.

Mitomycin-C

Mitomycin-C was originally isolated from cultures of *Streptomyces caespitosus* in Japan. The mechanism of action is uncertain but there are two main possibilities: firstly, mitomycin-C acts as an alkylating agent and forms cross-linkages with DNA, and, secondly, the drug generates free radicals.

The net result of these actions are alkylation, DNA strand breakage and inhibition of DNA and RNA synthesis.

Mitomycin-C is mainly used in the treatment of gastrointestinal carcinomas but has also been given as an intravesicular instillation for bladder cancer. The dose-limiting toxicity is delayed myelosuppression, with nadir white cell and platelet levels appearing 5 to 8 weeks after dosing. Nausea and vomiting occur in about a quarter of patients and diarrhoea is seen a little less frequently. Cumulative doses, in excess of 100mg, may lead to renal failure which is reversible if recognised soon enough, regular monitoring of renal function is, therefore, advisable. Pulmonary infiltration and fibrosis may develop but do not appear to be dose related.

Mitomycin-C is given by intravenous injection and causes painful cellulitis if it leaks outside the vein. Doses are usually of the order of 10mg per week.

Bleomycin

Bleomycin is a mixture of several glycopeptides derived from the fungus *Streptomyces verticillis* and was developed in Japan. The active peptides have a two-stage action, initially intercalating with DNA and then forming free radicals which cause fragmentation of the DNA chain with both single and double strand breaks. Bleomycin is of value in the treatment of testicular teratomas, lymphomas and some squamous cell carcinomas. It is also a useful agent for intracavitary administration to control malignant effusions.

In contrast to other cytotoxics, bleomycin causes little or no myelo-suppression. Pulmonary toxicity is, however, a major problem: initially manifest as a pneumonitis, it may progress to a fatal pulmonary fibrosis. This effect is dose related and is most frequently seen when the cumulative dose exceeds 300mg, although it has been reported with doses as low as 100mg. Underlying emphysema, an age of over 70 years and previous radiotherapy all increase the risk of lung damage. Patients who have received bleomycin also appear to have an increased risk of respiratory complications following anaesthetics. There is no specific therapy for bleomycin-induced lung damage and the changes are usually only partially reversible after stopping the drug. Skin toxicity is the other major side effect of the drug with dermatological changes seen in about 50 per cent of patients. These include: erythema, hyperkeratosis, peeling of the skin, brown pigmentation, the formation of bullae and ulceration. Painful hardening of the finger tips, alopecia, ridging of the nails and Raynaud's phenomenon may also occur. Transient fevers are quite often recorded for a few hours after injection of bleomycin.

Bleomycin may be given intramuscularly (with lignocaine to reduce discomfort), by intravenous injection or infusion or as an intracavitary instillation. Doses used range from 2 to 90mg.

Mithramycin

The value of mithramycin is limited by its severe toxicity and clinical indications are virtually restricted to second line treatment of testicular teratoma and management of refractory malignant hypercalcaemia. Its cytotoxic action is thought to result from binding to DNA but the details of this interaction are uncertain. Bone marrow suppression is the major toxicity with a particular tendency to thrombocytopenia. The resulting risk of haemorrhage is compounded by the fact that mithramycin may also interfere with blood clotting mechanisms. Gastrointestinal toxicity is common. Hepatotoxicity and serious renal damage have also been reported. Mithramycin is given intravenously at a dose of 25 microgrammes per kg daily for five days with courses repeated every 4 to 6 weeks.

Miscellaneous Compounds

Non-classical Alkylating Agents

*Cisplatin (Neoplatin, cis-*DDP) and Carboplatin (Paraplatin)

The development of these compounds stemmed from a chance observation, by Rosenberg in 1965, that an alternating current, delivered through platinum electrodes, inhibited the growth of bacteria in culture in a similar way to that seen with radiation or alkylating agents. It was subsequently found that platinum atoms from the electrodes entered the growth medium and formed complexes which arrested cell division. This led to the evaluation of cisplatin, a complex of chloride and ammonium ions with platinum, which has rapidly become established as a major cytotoxic drug with significant activity in a wide range of common solid tumours including testicular teratoma, ovarian carcinoma, bladder cancer and head and neck tumours. Cisplatin is, however, very toxic and a number of analogues have been developed with the object of retaining anticancer activity whilst reducing side effects. The first of these compounds to be generally available is carboplatin (Paraplatin).

Both cisplatin and carboplatin molecules carry a pair of chloride atoms which react with various components of DNA but, in particular, with the nitrogen at the N-7 position of guanine. The spatial arrangement of the platinum complexes is such that the two chlorines are able to react with different guanine moieties, thereby forming cross linkages. At first sight this appears similar to the mechanism of alkylating agents but, whereas they predominantly form cross linkages between paired strands of DNA (interstrand cross links), the platinum compounds also attach to bases on the same DNA chain (intrastrand linkages) (see Figure 3.6). The relative importance of inter- and intrastrand cross linkages in the cytotoxicity of platinum compounds remains uncertain and as intra-strand cross linkages are sometimes seen following therapy with classical alkylating agents, it may well be that, with time, the present distinction between platinum drugs and the classical alkylating agents will prove to be a semantic nicety rather than a genuine reflection of a difference in mechanisms of cytotoxicity.

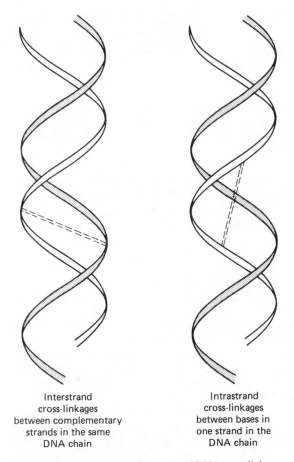

Interstrand
cross-linkages
between complementary
strands in the same
DNA chain

Intrastrand
cross-linkages
between bases in
one strand in the
DNA chain

Figure 3.6.   Interstrand and intrastrand DNA cross-linkages.

Cisplatin causes a degree of bone marrow suppression but gastrointestinal disturbance and renal damage are more major toxicities. The nausea and vomiting produced by cisplatin are intense and require supportive anti-emetic therapy for all patients (see Chapter 5). Renal toxicity occurs in about one-third of patients after a single dose of 50 to 75mg/m^2 but is usually mild and reversible. With further courses the incidence and severity of toxicity increases, with destruction of the renal tubules and, ultimately, irreversible renal failure may develop. Ensuring adequate renal function prior to treatment together with intensive intravenous hydration before, during and after cisplatin infusion reduces the risk of nephrotoxicity but greatly increases the complexity of drug administration. Cisplatin also interferes with renal tubular absorption of magnesium and tetany has occurred due to hypomagnesaemia during therapy. Ototoxicity with high frequency hearing loss, tinnitus and even deafness may occur, especially in older patients, and sensory peripheral neuropathy is a further potential complication. Given this toxicity profile it is not surprising that less toxic analogues of cisplatin have been sought. Carboplatin certainly carries significantly less risk of nephrotoxicity, neurotoxicity and ototoxicity. It is also generally less emetic than cisplatin. It does, however, produce a greater degree of bone marrow suppression and this is its dose limiting toxicity. Thrombocytopenia is more pronounced than leucopenia and may be slow to recover, necessitating intervals of 5 to 6 weeks between courses on occasions. Acute allergic reactions, with flushing, wheezing, tachycardia and hypotension, may occasionally occur within a few minutes of cisplatin or paraplatin administration. These respond to treatment with antihistamines or glucocorticoids.

Cisplatin is given by intravenous infusion, with appropriate pre- and post-hydration, and typical doses are 50–75mg/m^2. Carboplatin may be given without additional hydration, provided renal function is normal, and is usually administered as an intravenous infusion of 250–300mg/m^2.

Dacarbazine (DTIC, Imidazole Carboxamide)

This agent was originally synthesised, at the Southern Research Institute in the USA during the late 1950s, as a purine analogue which might act as an antimetabolite disturbing purine synthesis. Although the drug has found a limited clinical role in the treatment of Hodgkin's disease, malignant melanoma and soft tissue sarcomas, it is now considered that its antitumour activity is not related to inhibition of purine formation. Dacarbazine is metabolised to a number of compounds with alkylating activity and it is probable that its cytotoxicity is due to alkylation of DNA.

Principal toxic effects are bone marrow suppression and gastrointestinal disturbance. Alopecia and impairment of liver function have also been reported. Dacarbazine is given intravenously and a typical dose is 250–400mg/m^2.

Procarbazine (Natulan)

Procarbazine is derived from the hydrazines, which are one group of monoamine oxidase inhibitors widely employed in the treatment of depression. The discovery of procarbazine was a product of the search for new antidepressant drugs. Its precise mode of action remains unclear but alkylation and free radical formation have both been suggested.

Procarbazine is a useful drug in the management of Hodgkin's disease. Nausea and vomiting are the most marked side effects and bone marrow suppression is also seen. Procarbazine crosses the blood-brain barrier and is a mild monoamine oxidase inhibitor and its use may lead to somnolence, confusion and cerebellar ataxia. It should not be given with other monoamine oxidase inhibitors. The drug is given orally in doses ranging from 50 to 300mg daily.

Anthracenediones

Mitozantrone (Mitoxantrone, Novantrone)

Mitozantrone is a synthetic drug and is a member of a new class of compounds called the anthracenediones. These were derived from various chemical dyes. In fact the anthracenediones have a very similar structure to the anthracyclines, and mitozantrone is chemically similar to doxorubicin and its analogues. The mechanism of action of mitozantrone has still to be fully elucidated but certainly it intercalates with DNA and chelates some metals. Free radical formation, however, is less apparent than with the anthracyclines. Mitozantrone has demonstrated activity in breast cancer similar to that seen with doxorubicin and epirubicin and has also proved effective in lymphomas: its role in other tumours is still being explored.

Bone marrow suppression is the major toxicity of mitozantrone. As with the anthracyclines, nausea and vomiting, alopecia and cardiotoxicity occur but the frequency and severity of these side effects is less than that seen with doxorubicin. A typical dose schedule for single agent therapy is $12–14mg/m^2$ intravenously every 4 weeks.

Epipodophyllotoxins

Etoposide (Vepesid, VP16) and Teniposide (VM26)

These are semisynthetic derivatives of podophyllotoxin, which is a crystalline extract of the May Apple plant. Podophyllotoxin is known to bind to tubulin, in a similar manner to the vinca alkaloids, leading to metaphase arrest. Despite their close chemical similarity to podophyllotoxin, etoposide and teniposide do not affect microtubule formation but arrest replication in the premitotic phase of the cell cycle, during late G_2 and S, with subsequent appearance of single strand DNA breaks. The precise cause of these effects remains to be clarified. Etoposide has shown activity against a number of solid tumours, most notably small cell carcinoma of the bronchus and testicular teratoma. Teniposide is not commercially available in Britain but has shown activity against lymphomas and bladder cancer.

Bone marrow suppression is the dose limiting toxicity of both agents. Alopecia, nausea, vomiting, transient disturbance of liver enzymes and a mild peripheral neuropathy may also occur. Etoposide may be given orally or intravenously, a typical schedule being up to $300mg/m^2$ daily (by mouth) or $120mg/m^2$ daily (intravenously) for 5 days every 3–4 weeks. Teniposide is given intravenously at a dose of $30–40mg/m^2$ for 5 days every 2–4 weeks.

Hydroxyurea (Hydrea)

Hydroxyurea is an analogue of urea. It was first synthesised over 100 years ago and its ability to produce leucopenia in experimental animals was noted as long ago as the 1920s but it was not evaluated in cancer patients until the 1960s. It has subsequently found a place in tumour treatment, being of some value in chronic myeloid leukaemia, polycythaemia and choriocarcinoma.

It acts by inhibiting the ribonucleotide reductase enzyme system, thereby preventing DNA synthesis. Principal side effects of hydroxyurea include myelosuppression, nausea, vomiting and skin changes such as dryness, atrophy and erythema. The drug potentiates the effects of radiotherapy and may cause radiation recall phenomena with the development of redness or irritation in previously irradiated areas. It is given orally.

Amsacrine (Amsidine, AMSA)

Amsacrine is a synthetic member of the aminoacridine family of compounds. Its cytotoxicity is principally the result of its ability to intercalate with DNA. The drug has been evaluated in a wide range of tumours but has only shown significant activity in acute myeloid leukaemia and has been incorporated into a number of treatment regimes in this disease. Its main toxicity is myelosuppression, but mild nausea and vomiting also commonly occur. Alopecia, peripheral neuropathy, disturbed liver function and cardiotoxicity are occasional side effects, the latter being more likely if serum potassium levels are low. The drug is given intravenously.

Enzyme Therapy

Asparaginase

Chance observations during the 1950s led to the discovery that certain malignant cells were unable to synthesise asparagine and relied on the body pool for their supply of this essential amino acid. Asparaginase is an enzyme which splits asparagine into aspartic acid and ammonia; it can be obtained in large quantities from certain bacteria. The hope was that by giving the enzyme all free asparagine in the body would be destroyed, thereby depriving the tumour cells of an essential nutrient. The opportunity to exploit a biochemical difference between normal and malignant cells was exciting, but unfortunately for all its promise and theoretical importance the drug has proved disappointing in clinical practice and its usefulness is confined to remission induction in acute leukaemias.

Asparaginase is a toxic agent with a plethora of side effects including nausea, vomiting, hypersensitivity reactions and damage to the liver, kidneys, pancreas, central nervous system and clotting mechanisms.

Table 3.1. The pharmacology of cytotoxic drugs

Drug	Gastro-intestinal absorption	Plasma half-life	Degree of metabolism	Route of excretion of drug or active metabolites
Nitrogen mustard	Good[a]	10 min	Extensive	Bile+++ Urine+
Cyclophosphamide	Good	3–10 hr	Extensive	Bile++ Urine++
Ifosfamide	Good	4–6 hr	Partial	Urine+++ Bile+
Melphalan	Variable	2 hr	Extensive	Urine+++
Chlorambucil	Good	1½ hr	Extensive	Urine+++
Busulphan	Good	5 min	Extensive	Urine+++
Thiotepa	Unpredictable	3–4 hr	Extensive	Urine+++ Bile+
BCNU	Poor	6 min/68 min[c]	Extensive	Urine+++
CCNU	Good	None[b]	Extensive	Urine+++
Methyl-CCNU	Good	None[b]	Extensive	Urine+++
Methotrexate	Good	30 min/2–3 hrs/ 8–10 hrs[d]	Slight	Urine+++ Bile+
5-Fluorouracil	Variable	6–20 min	Extensive	Urine++ Lungs++
Cytosine arabinoside	Poor	12 min/3 hr[c]	Extensive	Urine+++
6-Mercaptopurine	Variable	50 min	Extensive	Urine+++
6-Thioguanine	Variable	90 min	Complete	Urine+++
Vincristine	Poor	1/7/160 min[d]	Extensive	Bile+++
Vinblastine	Variable	4 min/1 hr/20 hr[d]	Extensive	Bile+++
Vindesine	Poor	4 min/1½ hr/20 hr[d]	Extensive	Bile+++
Doxorubicin	None	15 min/5 hr/40 hr[d]	Extensive	Bile++ Urine++
Epirubicin	None	10 min/4 hrs/30 hrs[d]	Extensive	Bile+++ Urine+
Actinomycin-D	None	2 min	None	Bile+++ Urine+
Mitomycin-C	Good	15–30 min	Extensive	Urine+++
Bleomycin	None	20 min/4 hr[c]	Partial	Urine+++
Cisplatinum	None	45 min/20–80 hr[c]	Extensive	Urine+++ Bile+
Carboplatin	None	15 mins/3 hr[c]	Extensive	Urine+++ Bile+
Procarbazine	Good	10 min	Extensive	Urine+++
Dacarbazine	Good	3 hr	Uncertain	Urine+++
Mitozantrone	None	5 min/2 hr 10–200 hr[d]	Extensive	Bile+++ Urine+
Etoposide	Poor	30 min/3½ hr/ 25 hr[d]	Extensive	Urine+++
Asparaginase	None	14–22 hr	Extensive	

[a] Some uptake from gut but drug too corrosive to be given orally to humans.
[b] No drug detectable in plasma following oral administration.
[c] Biphasic half-title.
[d] Triphasic half-life.

Chapter 4

The Rationale of Cytotoxic Drug Therapy

Introduction

When cytotoxic drugs first became available for clinical use they opened up an entirely new field of medicine; as a consequence there was little or no guidance as to how the drugs should be used. As time went by results from clinical and laboratory studies provided some facts, and many theories, a number of which significantly influenced the development of chemotherapeutic practice. In this chapter the evolution of the use of cytotoxic drugs will be traced and those areas of research which have changed approaches to treatment, or given a theoretical basis for existing empirical techniques will be discussed. Initially, however, we need to remember some basic facts about tumour growth and kinetics which are relevant to cytotoxic therapy.

Tumour Regression and Cure

In spite of all the advances in cytotoxic therapy over the past 40 years, cure of cancer by drugs alone is possible in only a few relatively uncommon diseases. In recent years worthwhile remissions, with disappearance of all clinically detectable tumour, and complete relief of symptoms, have been achieved by cytotoxic therapy in a wide range of cancers, but the disease inevitably relapses and the patient finally dies. If cure is possible in a few conditions, and good remissions may be seen in many more, why is cancer not more frequently cured by drug therapy?

Consider an extremely simple kinetic model of a tumour which has a doubling time of three months and is made up solely of dividing cells. We know that such a tumour will not be clinically detectable until it contains a minimum of 10^9 cells and has a mass of about 1g. By the time the tumour cell population reaches 10^{12}, with a mass of about 1kg, the patient will be in a terminal state.

Normally in solid tumours the growth rate slows with increase in size, but for simplicity we will assume that this tumour has a constant growth rate. The time taken to increase in size from 10^9 to 10^{11} cells will be some 6–7 doubling times or 650–700 days. If the patient starts chemotherapy when the disease is advanced, as is usually the case, with the tumour cell population numbering 10^{11}, and treatment achieves a cell kill of three logs, then the tumour will be reduced from 10^{11} to 10^8 cells. The patient would have no clinically detectable tumour, and would *appear* to be cured. In fact there would still be over 100 million tumour cells remaining in the body and if these continued to grow at their original rate the tumour would regain its pretreatment size in 10 doublings or about 1000 days. So treatment will have induced a remission of three years' duration but will not have cured the tumour.

Animal experiments have shown that a single cancer cell inoculated into the body of a mouse can multiply to cause a lethal tumour. The therapeutic implication of this observation is that a cancer cannot be considered cured until the last malignant cell has been destroyed.

If a given cytotoxic drug, or combination of drugs, were able to achieve a 50 per cent tumour cell kill in two weeks this would be an exceptionally good result which, in practice, only occurs in a few rapidly dividing and highly sensitive tumours. If treatment was continued and this rate of cell kill maintained, then complete clinical remission (reduction of the tumour from 10^{11} to 10^8 cells) would be achieved in about 5 months. To cure the tumour, reducing the tumour cell population to zero, would require a further 14 months of therapy. Thus even this very responsive tumour would take one and a half years to cure. Based on this model the length of treatment for less sensitive, more slowly growing, lesions would extend to many years. In practice it is not possible to continue cytotoxic treatment for such long periods because of drug toxicity and the development of drug resistance by the tumour.

In those growths which are cured by drug treatment an additional factor has been suggested as well as extreme sensitivity to cytotoxics and a rapid mitotic rate: host immunity. It is postulated that immune mechanisms might be particularly active in these growths so that when chemotherapy has reduced the tumour cell population below a certain, unknown, critical level the body's own defences are able to destroy the remaining cancer cells.

Single Agent Continuous Therapy

When cytotoxic drugs were first introduced, the branch of therapeutics which appeared most similar to anticancer therapy was antimicrobial treatment, with the sulphonamides and antibiotics. The aim of treatment was the same in both instances – the eradication of a harmful cell population within the body – in the one case a bacterial population, in the other a tumour cell population.

The principles of antimicrobial chemotherapy were adopted by the early cancer chemotherapists and formed the basis of the technique known as single agent continuous cytotoxic therapy. The object of treatment was to maintain a near constant blood level of a single cytotoxic agent in the patient, until either unacceptable toxicity, drug resistance or cure resulted. Toxicity determined the amount of drug that could be given. As it was considered that the blood level of the drug should be as high as possible, the dose was adjusted upwards until toxicity was apparent and then maintained at a level which caused minimal side effects (such as slight nausea or a small depression in the white cell count).

This approach was based on the then accepted theory which stated that increase in tumour size was due to a far more rapid rate of cell division in malignant tissues than normal tissues. Thus, if a continuous blood level of a cytotoxic drug was maintained, there would be a toxic effect on normal cells. There would be a far more damaging effect on cancer cells because their much greater rate of mitosis would make them more susceptible to cytotoxic action. This theory of tumour growth is now known to be incorrect and, in almost every instance, the mitotic rate in tumours is far less than that in rapidly dividing normal tissues such as the bone marrow and gastrointestinal epithelium. Alternative explanations for cytotoxic activity had to be found and results from experiments looking at the relationship between dose and response provided some answers.

Fractional Cell Kill

In the mid-1960s Howard Skipper, in the USA, published the results of his studies on mice injected with L1210 leukaemia cells (Skipper HE et al., Cancer Treatment Reports, 35: 3–11, 1964 & 45: 5–28, 1965). From his experiments comes some of the fundamental scientific evidence on which contemporary chemotherapeutic practice is based. After first demonstrating the fact, referred to previously, that inoculation of a single L1210 cell could lead to the development of a fatal tumour, he went on to study the effects of chemotherapy on the pattern of growth of the leukaemia. On the basis of his findings he elaborated the following principles:

1. The per cent of varying size leukaemia cell populations killed by a given dose of a given drug was reasonably constant.

2. There is a close relationship between dosage level and the per cent of a given leukaemia cell population killed by an effective drug.

These results demonstrated that cytotoxic destruction of tumour cells follows first order kinetics, or fractional cell-kill, where a fixed *proportion* of susceptible cells will be destroyed by a given dose of drug during a specified period of time, not a fixed *number* of cells. For example, if a given dose of drug A kills 10 per cent of tumour cells then that dose will reduce a tumour cell population of 100 million to 90 million, but if there are only 10 cells in a tumour that same dose of drug will not result in cure, but will only reduce the number of cells from 10 to 9. The results also show that the greater the dose of drug given, the larger the fraction of cells killed.

These clear cut observations from animal tumour models are only partially reproducible in the clinical situation. There are numerous reasons for this but two particularly important factors should be mentioned: the kinetic heterogeneity and biochemical heterogeneity of human tumour cells.

Kinetic heterogeneity means that large tumour masses will contain a high proportion of slowly dividing, or non-dividing cells (in the G_0 phase of the cell cycle) and many cytotoxic agents are relatively ineffective against such cells. An initial reduction in the tumour cell population, brought about by surgery, radiotherapy or the use of specific cytotoxics active against G_0 cells (such as alkylating agents and anthracyclines) may well draw resting cells into the cell cycle, thereby increasing the proportion of dividing cells (a phenomenon known as "recruitment") and thus increasing the susceptibility of the tumour to subsequent doses of chemotherapy. In this way the proportion of cells killed could actually increase with further courses of treatment at the same dose, rather than remain constant.

This positive effect on cell-kill over a period of time is tempered by a negative effect due to biochemical variations in the cells. As will be seen later (Chapter 7) this aspect of tumour heterogeneity usually results in certain clones of cells being inherently resistant to the action of cytotoxics. Thus as treatment continues sensitive populations will be destroyed but the subpopulation of resistant cells survives and multiplies. As a result the fractional cell kill will tend to reduce with subsequent courses of treatment and the maximum response will be seen with the initial doses. This is the main reason why, however high the dose of drug used, single agent cytotoxic therapy very rarely results in tumour cure. It is also a major theoretical justification for giving cytotoxic drugs in combination rather than as single agents.

Combination Chemotherapy

In most branches of medicine it is considered good practice to use the minimum number of drugs possible to treat a given condition and this was an argument in favour of continuous single agent cytotoxic therapy. In the mid 1950s cancer research workers began to question this principle and argued that a combination of two cytotoxic agents would be more effective than a single drug.

The basis for this proposal is as follows. Cytotoxic drugs have a variety of actions on the dividing cell – an alkylating agent achieves its lethal effect by a completely different mechanism to an antimetabolite. Thus a tumour cell which may be resistant to one drug with a particular mode of action might well be susceptible to a different agent with an alternative form of cytotoxicity. Combining drugs with different mechanisms of cell-kill should therefore reduce the risk of encountering resistant cells and so increase fractional cell kill and improve response rates.

Initial animal experiments gave encouraging results with two drug therapy, or combination chemotherapy as it subsequently became known. Early clinical trials both in leukaemia and solid tumours confirmed the value of combination chemotherapy. In acute lymphatic leukaemia in children the median survival time prior to the introduction of chemotherapy was 5 months. The use of methotrexate as a single agent increased this to 9 months, and the initial combination of cyclophosphamide and vincristine resulted in another increase, to 14 months. Further refinements in combination regimes over the last twenty years now mean that more than 50 per cent of children with this disease are completely cured. Similarly in advanced breast cancer cyclophosphamide and 5-fluorouracil had proved two of the most effective single agents, producing remissions in about 25 per cent of patients but when the two drugs were combined the response rate rose to over 50 per cent.

In some instances combining two different agents has resulted in synergy – the results of treatment being better than would be expected from an additive effect of the two drugs used singly. For example, chlorambucil produces remissions in about 25 per cent of patients with Hodgkin's disease and similar results are obtained with vincristine. By combining the two drugs a 50 per cent remission rate could be anticipated but in fact the figure is closer to 65 per cent – the effect of the drugs in combination is greater than their combined single actions. Conversely a few drug combinations have proved antagonistic and certain drugs should not be used together (see Chapter 7).

After the initial use of two drug combination therapy the number of agents grouped together was increased to three and then to four, often with further improvement in results. For example, two drug treatment in Hodgkin's disease gave a remission rate of 65 per cent but use of four drugs (nitrogen mustard, procarbazine, prednisone and vincristine) increased this to 80 per cent. More recently protocols with as many as eight or ten different drugs have been reported and further successes in treatment claimed as a result of their application.

The initial two drug combinations were administered continuously with daily or twice weekly dosing. With the introduction of more intensive combinations severe toxicity was inevitable if the drugs were to be given continuously. The introduction of such regimes into clinical practice was only possible as a result of a complete rethinking of the basis for scheduling cytotoxic therapy.

Intermittent Chemotherapy

During the late 1950s and early 1960s laboratory studies identified a major difference between tumours and replicating normal tissues: the tumours had a diminished capacity for repair and repopulation after injury. Experiments showed that if a single dose of a cytotoxic drug was given then both normal and tumour cell populations would be reduced but the pre-treatment cell number would be regained much more rapidly in the normal tissue than the tumour.

These observations had major implications for scheduling of cytotoxic therapy. With continuous drug administration there is no opportunity for repair of drug-induced damage and hence no possibility of exploiting the difference in the repair capacities of normal and malignant tissues. If, however, the drug (or combination of drugs) is only given intermittently then the potential therapeutic advantages of this differential become apparent.

In order to see how altering the timing of drug administration can make use of differential recovery rates it is easiest to consider a simplified kinetic model of a tumour. The three factors determining growth rate are the rapidity of tumour cell division, the growth fraction and the cell loss factor. Let us assume that our theoretical tumour has a growth fraction of 100 per cent and zero cell loss. In such a tumour all the cells will be actively dividing and all the daughter cells will be capable of producing endless further generations of identical cells. This will result in exponential growth and if the log of the total cell number is plotted against unit time a straight line graph will result (as in Figure 4.1).

If a single cytotoxic treatment sufficient to reduce the tumour cell population by two logs is given, then the growth pattern will be that shown in Figure 4.2. Laboratory studies have indicated that tumour cells are not able to increase their rate of division following such damage and, as all the cells are dividing in our model tumour, no resting cells can be recruited to help in repopulation; thus the overall growth rate will be the same after treatment as it was before.

If we now consider the effect of such cytotoxic treatment on normal tissue as well (such as the bone marrow stem cell population) then we obtain the picture in Figure 4.3. The normal tissue population is diminished by the treatment but recovers initially far more rapidly than the malignant tissues. As the normal cell population approaches its pretreatment level homeostatic

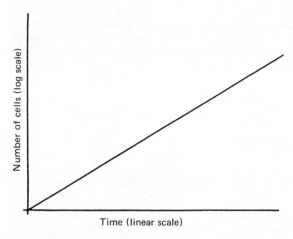

Figure 4.1. Exponential tumour growth.

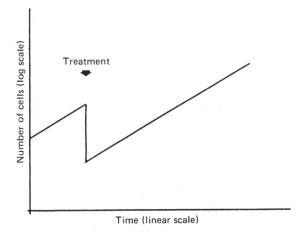

Figure 4.2. The effect of a single course of cytotoxic therapy on tumour growth.

mechanisms operate to slow the rate of proliferation but in almost every instance the restoration of the original cell number will be achieved more quickly in the normal tissue than its malignant counterpart.

If a series of treatments is given, with an interval for recovery of normal tissue between each treatment, it can be seen that, in theory, it is possible to eradicate the tumour without jeopardising the normal stem cell population (Figure 4.4). Treatment may be continued indefinitely without irreversible toxicity.

The time at which cytotoxic treatment is given is extremely important. If the interval between treatments is too short the normal stem cells will not have recovered sufficiently and cumulative toxicity will result, preventing adequate treatment (Figure 4.5). Similarly if the interval between courses is

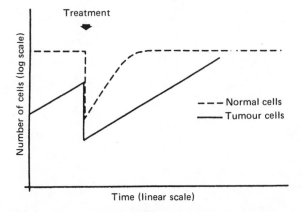

Figure 4.3. The effect of a single course of cytotoxic therapy on normal tissues.

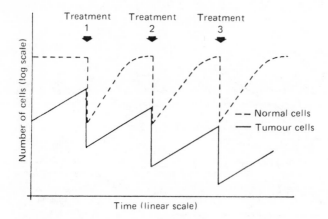

Figure 4.4. The effect of multiple courses of cytotoxic therapy on normal and tumour cell populations.

too long tumour cell recovery will be complete, allowing the tumour to remain static, or even increase in size, between treatments (Figure 4.6).

The splitting of cytotoxic treatment into short intensive intervals is known as intermittent, or pulsed, chemotherapy and has allowed multiple drug combinations to be used without causing irreversible toxicity, with a consequent increase in response rates. The theoretical advantages of intermittent therapy compared to continuous drug administration may be summarised as follows:

1. Intermittent therapy allows maximum exploitation of the differential in recovery times between normal and malignant tissues, leading to maximum tumour cell kill with minimum toxicity.

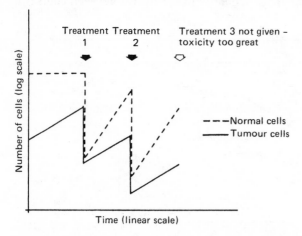

Figure 4.5. The effect of multiple courses of cytotoxic therapy with too short an interval for normal cell recovery.

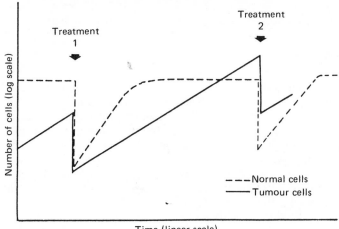

Figure 4.6. Multiple courses of cytotoxic therapy with too long an interval, allowing increases in tumour cell population between courses.

2. This relative lack of toxicity allows intermittent therapy to be continued for much longer periods than continuous treatment and thereby increases the chance of cure.

3. Pulsing of treatment allows higher doses of individual drugs, or combinations of drugs, to be given during each treatment course than would be possible with continuous therapy. As the percentage cell kill is proportional to the dose of drug given (see above) then this increase in dose should result in a greater reduction in the tumour cell population.

4. Recovery of normal tissue between treatments includes restoration of the immune system, which is not possible with continuous therapy, and immune mechanisms may be important in destroying small tumour cell populations.

Figure 4.3 demonstrates how intermittent combination chemotherapy has the potential for tumour cure but the great majority of cancers are not eradicated by such treatment. A number of factors influence the sensitivity of individual tumours to this approach, including the scheduling of therapy, tumour growth fraction, drug access to the tumour and drug resistance.

Scheduling of Therapy

Figures 4.4 and 4.5 clearly demonstrate the importance of timing in drug administration. As yet there is no method of determining optimum treatment schedules for individual tumours. Current protocols offer guidance for drug administration in specific types of tumour, based on clinical and experimental observations, but these are essentially generalisations and will not represent the optimum schedule for each and every cancer of that particular type.

Tumour Growth Fraction

Growth fractions in human tumours vary greatly; they are highest in the acute leukaemias and lymphomas but fall to levels of 10 per cent or less in many solid tumours. Dividing cells are much more sensitive to the effects of cytotoxics than resting cells and hence the growth fraction reflects the proportion of the tumour cell population susceptible to cytotoxic action: the response to chemotherapy is dependent on the growth fraction. As we have seen, the phenomenon of recruitment may increase the growth fraction during treatment but even so it is unlikely that growth fractions of 90 to 100 per cent are ever achieved with most solid tumours.

Drug Access

One reason for the difference in growth fraction betwen solid tumours and leukaemias is anoxia. Leukaemias and lymphomas generally exist in a well vascularised environment which means that the tumour cells are well oxygenated. In solid tumours the cells are packed tightly together and areas of hypoxia and necrosis are common. Experiments have shown that the growth fraction is dramatically reduced in these anoxic areas. Such areas of anoxia develop because of an inadequate blood supply and it therefore follows that cytotoxic drugs, which are carried in the blood, will have little chance of reaching these necrotic sites, where some viable tumour cells will still be present. This is an additional, anatomical, factor which helps explain the poor response to chemotherapy of most solid tumours.

Drug Resistance

As has been described a proportion of the cells in any tumour may be inherently resistant to the drug, or drugs, being used against them and this proportion will vary from tumour to tumour.

Developments in cytotoxic administration over the last twenty years have been aimed at overcoming these problems and four complementary avenues of research have looked at the timing of drug administration, the choice of drugs for combination chemotherapy, the dose of drug that should be given and drug toxicity.

Timing of Cytotoxic Therapy

Adjuvant Therapy

So far we have established that there is a strong argument for splitting cytotoxic treatment into a number of short pulses followed by recovery intervals, but nothing has been said about the timing of treatment in relation to the natural history of the disease. Initially the use of cytotoxic drugs was almost exclusively restricted to the treatment of advanced cancer, being used as a last resort when more conventional methods, such as surgery and radiotherapy, had failed. By the mid 1970s, however, a case could be made for using chemotherapy as an adjunct to surgery, or irradiation, in the primary management of certain cancers. The theoretical basis for this approach, which has become known as adjuvant therapy, derived from a number of experimental observations, may be summarised as follows:

1. As a tumour grows the growth fraction decreases, resulting in progressive slowing of growth.

2. As a tumour grows the blood supply to many areas diminishes and the cells furthest from the capillaries become increasingly hypoxic. These hypoxic cells are less likely to divide and are less likely to receive adequate concentrations of cytotoxics than those with a better blood supply.

3. The longer a tumour is allowed to grow the greater the chance of spontaneous cell mutations which might result in drug resistance.

The converse of these observations is that the younger the tumour the greater the growth fraction, the greater the oxygenation of the tumour cells and the less probable that resistant cells have developed. These three factors all increase the sensitivity of the tumour to chemotherapy. Therefore it may be argued that the younger the tumour the more likely it is to be cured by cytotoxic treatment.

By the time a solid cancer is clinically detectable it is almost certainly beyond cure by cytotoxics alone (with a few uncommon exceptions). There are, however, a number of tumours where the primary lesion may be easily destroyed by surgery or irradiation but the condition will subsequently prove fatal because of microscopic metastases which were present, but clinically undetectable, at the time of primary treatment. Immediately after primary treatment the tumour cell population in these patients will be relatively small. Traditionally no further treatment would be given to these patients until metastases became clinically apparent and these would then be treated palliatively, all hope of cure having been abandoned.

The rationale of adjuvant therapy is to treat patients who are thought to be at risk of harbouring occult metastases with cytotoxic drugs at the time of their initial surgery or radiation, rather than waiting until clinical recurrence is apparent. In this way an attempt is made to destroy residual or metastatic tumour cell populations when they are at their smallest and hence, for the reasons outlined above, at their most vulnerable.

Adjuvant therapy has been applied with considerable success in some paediatric cancers but, with the possible exception of breast cancer, has still to make a significant impact on common adult malignancies.

Neo-adjuvant Therapy

Adjuvant chemotherapy has usually been given following initial surgery or irradiation, but recently it has been suggested that cytotoxic treatment might be given prior to ablation of the primary tumour. This concept has been termed neo-adjuvant therapy and it is argued that it offers advantages for control of both the primary tumour and any micrometastases that may be present.

Potential benefits in the control of the primary include tumour shrinkage, which will make complete surgical removal both easier and more certain, or, if radiotherapy is to be given, will improve the vascularity and hence the oxygenation of the residual tumour mass, thereby increasing the chance of successful irradiation (since hypoxic cells are radio-resistant). In addition the response of the primary will act as an *in vivo* sensitivity test for chemotherapy so that if primary tumour shrinkage is seen with neo-adjuvant treatment this would indicate that the cancer is susceptible to the given drugs and that these should be continued after surgery, or radiotherapy, as conventional adjuvant therapy to ensure the destruction of micrometastases.

Potential benefits for the control of micrometastases result from the fact that neo-adjuvant therapy is given earlier than adjuvant therapy, which may on occasions be delayed for several weeks, or months, if there are complications following initial surgery or irradiation. The theoretical advantages of starting systemic therapy sooner are that as time progresses the growth fraction decreases and the likelihood of resistant cells appearing increases, so that the earlier treatment is given the more susceptible the micrometastases will be to its effects. There are also laboratory data suggesting that when a primary tumour is removed the growth rate of micrometastases is actually enhanced. Whether this applies in human tumours is not known but the observation has been used as a further argument in support of neo-adjuvant therapy, since it might inhibit such growth enhancement.

The major disadvantage of this approach is that not all tumours will be sensitive to the given drugs so that, in many instances, neo-adjuvant therapy will not only be ineffective but also harmful in that it will delay definitive treatment and expose the patients to unnecessary drug toxicity. At present preliminary clinical studies have suggested some benefit from neo-adjuvant treatment in head and neck cancer, carcinoma of the cervix and osteogenic sarcoma. Definitive trials are under way to establish whether there is a place for neo-adjuvant therapy in routine practice.

Choice of Drugs for Combination Chemotherapy

The principles underlying the choice of drugs for combination chemotherapy are a matter of common sense and may be stated as follows:

1. All drugs in the combination should be of proven value in the disease they are intended to treat.

2. The drugs should have different modes of cytotoxic action.

3. If possible the dose limiting toxicities of the chosen agents should be different so that additive toxicity does not limit the dose intensity of treatment.

Adherence to these simple guidelines has resulted in the major successes seen with combination chemotherapy over the past twenty years. During that time two further concepts have been promoted to guide drug selection: consideration of the effect of individual agents on the cell cycle and the use of alternating non-cross·resistant regimes. Although the value of these approaches remains uncertain the rationale for their use should be described as they are often discussed.

Cytotoxic Drugs and the Cell Cycle

Experiments during the 1960s showed that the pattern of cell kill following cytotoxic treatment of lymphoma cells varied with the different drugs used. All the agents tested fell into one of three groups and the different results could be related to the cell cycle. The first pattern of response was similar to that seen with radiotherapy in that cells at all stages of the cell cycle together with resting cells in G_0 were destroyed. In the next group the drugs had no effect on G_0 cells but those at all other stages of the cycle were affected. The drugs in the last group only affected cells at specific parts of the cell cycle whilst at other stages in the cycle the cells were relatively resistant. Agents in the first two groups have been termed cycle-specific whereas those in the last group are known as phase-specific. Table 4.1 lists some of the drugs in each category.

Table 4.1.   Examples of phase-specific and cycle-specific cytotoxic drugs

Cycle-specific agents	Phase-specific agents
Nitrogen mustard	Methotrexate
Cyclophosphamide	Cytosine arabinoside
Melphalan	6-Mercaptopurine
Chlorambucil	6-Thioguanine
Busulphan	Vincristine
Thiotepa	Vinblastine
Nitrosoureas	Vindesine
5-Fluorouracil	Bleomycin
Doxorubicin	Procarbazine
Daunorubicin	Etoposide
Actinomycin-D	Teniposide
Mitomycin-C	Hydroxyurea
Dacarbazine	

These observations led to increasing interest in the concepts of synchrony and recruitment in relation to drug selection and scheduling. At any one time dividing cells in a tumour are at various stages of the cell cycle and if a phase-specific agent was administered only a fraction of the cancer cells would be in the susceptible phase of the cycle. In theory, however, cell kill could be maximised by blocking the cell cycle, with a drug such as vincristine, until all the dividing cells were held at the same point and then, having synchronised the proliferating population, removing the blocking agent and after a suitable interval giving an appropriate phase-specific agent. All the dividing cells would simultaneously enter the phase at which the drug was active and maximum cell kill would be achieved. Interest in recruitment was based on the theory that if all the actively dividing cells in a tumour could be destroyed by a course of treatment with a cycle specific agent then the resting cells would be drawn into the cell cycle and would be vulnerable to a subsequent course of treatment with a phase-specific drug. Two major practical difficulties with these techniques are the problem of precise scheduling for individual tumours and the likelihood that normal cell populations will also be synchronised, or recruited, thus compounding toxicity. Nevertheless during the 1970s many, often highly complex, "kinetic" schedules for combination therapy were devised to try and take advantage of the difference between phase and cycle-specific drugs. Although a number of these regimes were clinically active there is no evidence that any of them were superior to more conventional combination chemotherapy protocols.

Alternating Non-cross Resistant Regimes

In many instances an initial response to combination chemotherapy will ultimately be followed by relapse, with recurrence of the original tumour. As we have seen, drug resistance is considered a major cause of such treatment failures: the cytotoxic combination kills the sensitive cells but the resistant cells survive and eventually repopulate the tumour. Clearly the chances of drug resistance will be reduced by using an increased number of non-cross resistant drugs with different modes of cell kill. To avoid undue toxicity the combinations are then split into two separate regimes given in alternating courses. The classic example of this approach is the use of two combinations MOPP (nitrogen Mustard, vincristine [Oncovin], prednisolone and procarbazine) and ABVD (doxurubicin [Adriamycin], bleomycin, vinblastine and Dacarbazine) which have been used in alternating cycles in the treatment of Hodgkin's disease. Improved response rates have been seen as a result but it is not clear whether response duration and overall survival will be enhanced. Certainly similar attempts to use alternating regimes in breast and lung cancer have not resulted in any increase in survival.

An alternative application of this approach has been to use an initial combination to induce a remission and then to give a non-cross-resistant regime as maintenance therapy thereafter. This approach has proved beneficial in acute lymphatic leukaemia in children but has not shown any benefit in adult solid tumours.

Drug Dose

Experiments in the 1960s suggested that only 20 per cent of stem cell are actively dividing in the bone marrow at any one time, the remaining 80 per cent being in the G_0 phase. Further studies suggested that if the dividing marrow stem cells were reduced by cytotoxic therapy then it took some 4 days for the remaining stem cells to move from G_0 into active division. The implication of these observations was that for a period of 3–4 days high doses of cytotoxics could be given as only 20 per cent of the marrow stem cell population would be affected during this time, leaving a more than adequate reserve of resting cells for subsequent repopulation. From Skipper's original experiments, one would expect that the higher the dose of cytotoxic given the greater the tumour cell kill. These two sets of laboratory data formed the rationale for high dose cytotoxic therapy which was extensively evaluated during the 1970s. Methotrexate was the favoured agent for these studies as its toxicity could be arrested at any time by the administration of leucovorin (see Chapter 5). Protocols in a number of tumours introduced ultra-high doses of methotrexate, together with leucovorin rescue 24–48 hours later. Responses were seen but, as time passed, there was increasing uncertainty as to whether the results really were any better than those seen with other combinations and this lack of definite evidence of superiority, coupled with the inconvenience and expense of the technique has meant that, with the exception of treatment of osteogenic sarcoma, high-dose methotrexate therapy is now seldom used.

Improvement in bone marrow transplantation techniques during the 1970s offered another option for high-dose therapy. The basis for this was that if marrow could be provided by a matched donor, or obtained from the patient prior to treatment, high-dose chemotherapy could then be given at levels which would completely ablate the remaining marrow but the patient could be rescued by infusions of their own, or the donor's, stored marrow cells. Once again the success of the technique has been limited, partly because of dose-limiting toxicity to other organs and also the difficulty in repeating courses due to the limited marrow reserves available for reinfusion. Although, occasionally, dramatic responses have been reported there is no clear evidence that such treatment has improved overall survival in any tumour. This technique should not be confused with the use of radiation and high-dose chemotherapy to destroy leukaemic bone marrow prior to infusion of normal healthy marrow from matched donors (see Chapter 15).

In the past few years increasing attention has been focussed on the actual doses given in combination regimes. Although for many tumours oncologists will tend to use identical combinations of drugs the precise dose, timing and duration of therapy may vary considerably. These variables have been grouped together in the concept of dose-intensity which is a measure of the total dose of a drug, or combination of drugs, given in unit times. Retrospective surveys looking at the combination of cyclophosphamide, methotrexate and 5-fluorouracil in breast cancer and 5-fluorouracil as a single agent in large bowel carcinoma have suggested that dose-intensity is important, with a clear correlation between increasing dose-intensity and increased response rates. Similar analyses in lung cancer have, however, failed to show any improvement in response or survival as a result of increased dose-intensity.

At this point in time the importance of dose-intensity remains unclear. Animal tumour models show a definite relationship between increased dose and increased cell kill but, as we have seen, factors such as drug resistance and kinetic heterogeneity make this relationship less certain in human cancers. Also the clinical analyses advocating increased dose-intensity have all been retrospective and, as such, are inherently inaccurate. Only when the results of prospective randomised clinical trials are available comparing different dose-intensities of the same regime in the same tumour type will this question be answered.

Reduced Toxicity

During the 1970s the success of combination chemotherapy in conditions such as Hodgkin's disease and testicular teratoma led to increasingly aggressive regimes being employed in a wide range of advanced cancers. By the early 1980s, however, it was apparent that such intensive treatment seldom significantly improved results and all too often was accompanied by severe toxicity. As a consequence there has been a growing trend to devise drug schedules which maintain the response rates seen with such intensive regimes but which cause substantially fewer and less severe side effects. This movement has been fuelled by the development of a number of analogues of existing cytotoxic agents which are claimed to retain the efficacy of their parent compounds but to cause significantly less toxicity.

Continuous Infusion Chemotherapy

Another approach that has been introduced in recent years in the hope of reducing toxicity has been continuous infusion chemotherapy. The development of implantable venous catheters and portable infusion pumps (see Chapter 5) over the last ten years has meant that that cytotoxics may be continuously infused over periods of weeks or even months, allowing prolonged constant plasma concentrations of the drug to be maintained. The theoretical advantages of this are:

1. Regardless of the length of the cell cycle of individual tumour cells the cytotoxic would always be present when a sensitive phase of the cycle was reached.

2. The transport of cytotoxics across tumour cell membranes may depend not only on drug concentration but on the time for which the drug is available to the cell membrane, in which case continuous infusion would enhance drug uptake by malignant cells.

3. Many cytotoxics have short pharmacological half-lives (see Table 3.1) and such agents may be more effective if exposed to the tumour cell for prolonged periods rather than given by intermittent bolus injections.

4. When given continuously the concentration of drug in the plasma is far lower than the levels seen immediately after bolus injections or short infusions: therefore many of the acute toxicities of the drug may be avoided.

Conversely it could be argued that normal cells will also suffer prolonged exposure to the drug, with a consequent increase in toxicity, and that the concentration of drug during continuous infusion may be too low to be effective. Nonetheless continuous infusion has been employed with a number of different agents. For many it has proved either ineffective or toxic but for a number of drugs, including doxorubicin, bleomycin, 5-fluorouracil, ifosfamide and the vinca alkaloids, initial results suggest that toxicity may be substantially reduced whilst efficacy is retained. Randomised studies are needed, however, to determine whether this approach is actually superior to more conventional administration.

These attempts to minimise side effects are not without their critics who argue that to concentrate efforts on reducing toxicity is a negative attitude, with a tacit acceptance that present response rates cannot be improved, and that increases in survival and cure will only occur by pursuing a more aggressive attitude to treatment. It may be, however, that by devising better tolerated schedules patient compliance will be improved and total drug doses might actually be increased with a consequent improvement in response rates.

Chapter 5

The Management of the Side Effects of Cytotoxic Drugs

Introduction

The ability of cytotoxic drugs to cure malignant disease is limited by two factors, drug resistance of tumour cells and the toxic effects of treatment on normal tissues. A number of techniques have been developed in an attempt to overcome the problems created by drug toxicity, in the hope of allowing higher doses of cytotoxics to be given, thereby increasing the chance of cure. Before considering the prevention and management of specific side effects it is important to realise that the very considerable hazards involved in the use of cytotoxic agents may be minimised by taking a few routine precautions.

Routine Precautions

It is essential to know, before treatment is started, what side effects might occur with a given drug or combination. With this knowledge appropriate monitoring of the patient may be arranged so that side effects are detected promptly and treatment may be stopped, or supportive measures introduced, before severe or irreversible toxicity develops. For this reason cytotoxic drugs should only be administered by clinicians with special expertise in oncology who are experienced in this therapeutic area. When all the drugs involved have potentially lethal toxicity, the use of cancer chemotherapy must be recognised as a specialised area of medical practice and restricted to those doctors with expert knowledge of the subject.

Numerous studies in many different types of cancer have consistently demonstrated that the better the general condition of the patient the greater the chance of a response to treatment and the better the tolerance of any side effects from such treatment. It is therefore important that before cytotoxics are given the patient's overall physical condition is as good as possible, with particular attention being paid to such factors as correcting anaemia, eradicating infection and ensuring the best possible nutritional status for the individual patient.

Before starting cytotoxic therapy all patients should have a full blood count and biochemical investigations, including tests of renal and liver function. Critical values for white cell and platelet counts vary with different clinical situations, but in general patients with a white cell count below 3,000 per mm^3, or a platelet count below 100,000 per mm^3 should not be given myelosuppressive cytotoxics. Many cytotoxics are either metabolised in the liver or excreted unchanged in the urine (see Table 3.1). Impaired hepatic or renal function means that high concentrations of these drugs remain in the circulation for much longer than normal which will result in excessive toxicity. Therefore if there is clinical or biochemical evidence of renal or hepatic dysfunction drugs which require either site for their metabolism or excretion should be avoided or given at reduced doses, the precise level of dose reduction being, once again, a matter of judgement based on experience.

One specific side effect which may be avoided by careful patient selection is the encephalopathy caused by ifosfamide. An analysis of women with cervical cancer who received the drug showed that a low serum albumin, a raised serum creatinine and the presence of pelvic tumour greatly increased the risk of neurotoxicity. Thus by selecting only those patients with normal albumin and creatinine levels, who have no gross pelvic malignancy, for ifosfamide therapy the likelihood of neurological complications is dramatically reduced.

Bone Marrow Toxicity

Nearly all cytotoxics cause bone marrow suppression at therapeutic doses but, as was seen in Chapter 2, the severity and duration of myelosuppression varies considerably with different agents. The nadir of myelosuppression occurs 7 to 14 days after administration of most drugs with a return to pretreatment levels over the next one to two weeks. A few drugs, including the nitrosoureas, mitozantrone, mitomycin-C and procarbazine, cause delayed myelosuppression with nadir levels appearing 28 to 42 days after treatment and recovery taking anything up to another 3 to 4 weeks.

Leucopenia

The most frequent manifestation of cytotoxic-induced bone marrow toxicity is leucopenia. The main hazard associated with leucopenia is increased susceptibility to infection. Provided the nadir leukocyte count remains above 1,000 per mm^3 the chance of developing severe infective complications is small and no specific action is required. If the leukocyte count falls much below 1,000 per mm^3 the risk of infection increases considerably, especially if the nadir persists for more than 5 days. In these circumstances a number of broad-spectrum antibiotic regimes have been recommended in order to prevent infection. These usually include combinations of carbenicillin with an amino-glycoside, such as gentamycin, and a cephalosporin.

An alternative form of prophylaxis against infection is the use of protected environments. These are sterile rooms with laminar air flow systems consisting of independent air-conditioning pumping air through microbial filters into the room at positive pressure in order to create a sterile atmosphere. The patient is then isolated in the room. Two-way cupboards provide access for sterilised bed linen and clothing and also for food, which has been passed through microwave and infra-red ovens to destroy bacteria. These sterile wards are expensive to construct and maintain and a smaller portable version has been devised. This consists of a large, plastic, air-tight tent, which encloses the patient's bed and is connected to an air-conditioning system supplying micro-organism-free air. Such small "life-islands" add the sensation of claustrophobia to the feeling of isolation experienced by patients in the larger sterile rooms.

A further problem is the risk of infection presented by the patient himself. Bacteria or fungi normally present on the skin or in the bowel may become pathogenic when the white cell count is very low and so they must be eradicated. This involves showering, disinfection, the application of topical antibiotics to body orifices and oral non-absorbable antibiotics, such as neomycin, to sterilise the bowel. Protected environments do reduce the incidence of infection but the expense, the psychological problems associated with isolation of the patient and the vigorous measures necessary to maintain a pathogen-free environment mean that these units are only used for those who are severely neutropenic, for example those who are having their marrow ablated by radiation and cytotoxics prior to bone marrow transplantation.

Granulocyte transfusions are sometimes given to patients who are leukopenic and develop an infection which fails to respond to antibiotics within 48 to 72 hours, particularly if the granulocyte count falls below 200 per mm^3. Such transfusions are prepared either by centrifugation of pooled blood from a number of donors or continuous filtration (leukopharesis) of blood from a single donor. The cells are given within 24 hours of harvesting and transfusions are usually repeated daily. The increase in circulating white cell levels varies enormously after such transfusions. These variations have led many experts to question whether such transfusions are really beneficial, and at this time the value of granulocyte transfusion is still debated.

Thrombocytopenia

Severe thrombocytopenia due to cytotoxic therapy is less common than leukopenia. Transient profound falls in the platelet count to levels of 30,000 to 50,000 per mm^3, which might be sufficient to cause bruising or spontaneous skin haemorrhages (petechiae) may usually be managed with small doses of corticosteroids. If the platelet count falls below 20,000 per mm^3 or if more severe bleeding occurs then transfusion of platelet concentrates is indicated. These are prepared in a similar way to the granulocyte transfusions. On average each 500ml unit of platelet rich plasma will increase the platelet count by 5,000 to 7,000 per mm^3 for each square metre of body surface area. When used prophylactically sufficient platelets should be given to raise the count above 20,000 per mm^3, but if active bleeding is present then levels of 50,000 to 80,000 per mm^3 will be needed in order to achieve haemostasis. Depending on the severity of thrombocytopenia and the presence of complications such as infection or bleeding, transfusions will be necessary every 1 to 3 days.

Anaemia

As explained in Chapter 2, anaemia sufficient to necessitate blood transfusion is seldom seen as a result of cytotoxic therapy. If a patient receiving chemotherapy is found to have a falling haemoglobin with the level going below 10g/dl then other causes for the anaemia, such as occult blood loss or haemolysis, must be vigorously excluded before the condition is attributed to cytotoxic treatment.

Nausea and Vomiting

Although nausea and vomiting are often very distressing side effects of chemotherapy the ability of individual cytotoxics to cause emesis varies considerably. Commonly used drugs may therefore be broadly classified into three groups, depending on whether sickness is likely to be mild, moderate or severe following their administration at standard doses (Table 5.1). The use of two or more emetogenic agents in combination will obviously increase the likelihood and severity of symptoms.

The principal agents used to counteract cytotoxic-induced emesis are shown in Table 5.2, together with their main site(s) of action and typical dose schedules. During the 1960s and early 1970s phenothiazines and subsequently

Table 5.1. The degree of emesis caused by individual cytotoxic drugs when given at standard doses

Severe emesis	Moderate emesis	Mild emesis
Nitrogen mustard	Cyclophosphamide[a,b]	Chlorambucil
Actinomycin-D	Ifosfamide	5-Fluorouracil
Doxorubicin[b]	Melphalan[a]	Vincristine
Dacarbazine	Nitrosoureas	Vinblastine
Cisplatinum	Methotrexate[a]	Vindesine
	Cytosine arabinoside[a]	Bleomycin
	Epirubicin[b]	Mitozantrone
	Mitomycin-C	Amsacrine
	Procarbazine	
	Carboplatin	
	Etoposide	

[a] Drug is sometimes given at higher doses with increased severity of symptoms.
[b] Drug is sometimes given at lower doses with reduced severity of symptoms.

Table 5.2. Principal anti-emetic agents used in cancer chemotherapy

Anti-emetic	Site of action	Typical dose schedule
Dopamine antagonists		
Metoclopramide	Inhibits dopamine receptors in chemoreceptor trigger zone (CTZ) and 5HT$_3$ receptors in small bowel	Low dose: 10–20mg po iv 8 hrly. High dose: up to 10mg/kg iv in 24 hours.
Domperidone	Inhibits dopamine receptors in CTZ	10–20mg 4–8 hrly po or 60mg 4–8 hrly pr
Cannabinoids		
Tetrahydro-cannabinol	Inhibits vomiting centre	5–15mg po 4 hrly
Nabilone	Inhibits vomiting centre	1–2mg po 12 hrly
Levonantrodol	Inhibits vomiting centre	1–2mg po/im 4 hrly
Corticosteroids		
Dexamethasone	Unknown	16–60mg po/iv daily
Phenothiazines		
Prochlorperazine	Inhibits dopamine receptors in CTZ	5–10mgs po/iv/im/pr 8 hrly
Chlorpromazine	Inhibits dopamine receptors in CTZ	25mg po/im/iv 8 hrly
Butyrophenones		
Haloperidol	Inhibits dopamine receptors in CTZ	1–2mg po/iv 3–6 hrly
Benzodiazepines		
Lorazepam	Effect on higher cerebral centres	2–4mg po 4 hrly
5HT$_3$ antagonists		
GR38032F	Inhibits 5HT$_3$ receptors in small bowel	4–8mg po/iv 6 hrly

metoclopramide formed the mainstay of anti-emetic therapy and were reasonably effective against those agents causing mild or moderate sickness. The introduction of doxorubicin into combination regimes in the mid-1970s and the profound nausea and vomiting produced by cisplatin, which became available in the late 1970s, caused symptoms which the agents in Table 5.2, given at conventional doses, were unable to control.

High-dose metoclopramide therapy was introduced in the early 1980s in order to combat severe sickness. This certainly improved control but was associated with a significant incidence of neurotoxicity, in particular extra-pyramidal reactions, comprising increase in muscle tone, spasm of the facial muscles, trismus, difficulty with speech and other disturbing symptoms. As a result domperidone was introduced in the hope that it would retain the anti-emetic activity of metoclopramide without its CNS toxicity. Unfortunately, however, when given at high doses occasional severe cardiac side effects were seen which precluded further use of this approach, although the drug when given at conventional doses of 10 to 20mg tds remains a useful alternative for control of mild or moderate emesis.

The cannabinoids were developed as a further therapeutic option but proved relatively ineffective in the control of severe nausea and were associated with troublesome hallucinatory side effects. Although the latter were reduced when the drugs were combined with phenothiazines, emetic control was not greatly improved.

During the early 1980s dexamethasone and lorazepam were both demonstrated to have anti-emetic activity. Although neither agent was effective alone in controlling severe emesis the euphoriant effect of the steroid and the sedative and amnesic properties of lorazepam introduced additional aspects to symptom control which increased patient tolerance of chemotherapy-induced sickness. As a result there has been an increasing tendency to use these agents in combination with other anti-emetics, usually high-dose metoclopramide, for the control of severe nausea and vomiting. There is now good evidence that these combinations are more effective than high-dose metoclopramide alone.

The latest development is the introduction of $5HT_3$-receptor antagonists. As yet these drugs are still undergoing evaluation but early results suggest they are highly effective in the control of cisplatin-induced emesis and in the prevention of severe sickness due to intensive combination chemotherapy with other drugs. They also seem remarkably free from side effects. If their initial promise is sustained they could well completely alter the current patterns of management of cytotoxic-induced emesis.

Anticipatory nausea and vomiting is a particular problem which often proves extremely difficult to control. It is defined as sickness occurring before, and in anticipation of, chemotherapy administration and the longer treatment continues the greater the risk of its appearance. Undoubtedly experiencing moderate or severe sickness in the early stages of treatment predisposes to its development and a major factor in its prevention is ensuring good control, or better still complete avoidance, of emetic symptoms from the outset of chemotherapy. More specifically the use of lorazepam, with its amnesic effect, probably helps to reduce the likelihood of anticipatory emesis developing, particularly in those patients who will be given drugs, or combinations, which might result in severe sickness.

Alopecia

Alopecia is not a life-threatening complication of cytotoxic therapy but for many patients the fact that they may lose their hair is the most distressing aspect of treatment. Attempts have been made to overcome this problem by reducing the blood supply to the hair follicles during drug administration by using either scalp tourniquets or scalp cooling.

The most widely used scalp tourniquet is a modified blood pressure cuff, about 5 centimetres wide, which is placed around the head just below the hair line, and then connected to a sphygmomanometer. The pressure in the cuff is then raised to some 20 mm of mercury above systolic blood pressure and the cytotoxic injection given. The cuff is left in place for 20 to 30 minutes following the injection, before pressure is reduced. The use of scalp tourniquets is controversial and although they certainly delay the onset of alopecia it is still not certain that the overall incidence of hair loss is reduced.

The use of ice packs or commercially available "cold caps" and "ice turbans" can reduce the scalp temperature below 25°C within 10 minutes; this results in extreme vasoconstriction of the skin capillaries with a consequent reduction in blood supply to the hair follicles. These scalp cooling measures have been widely used to control epilation resulting from doxorubicin administration. They are certainly effective with doses below 50mg per m^2 but their value at higher doses is less certain.

Both tourniquets and cooling are relatively uncomfortable procedures and can usually only be tolerated for 20 to 30 minutes after drug administration. They are, therefore, not suitable for patients receiving drugs by prolonged infusion, nor are they effective for agents with active plasma half-lives of more than 15 to 20 minutes or in patients with impaired liver function when metabolism of the drug may be delayed. These techniques should not be used for patients at risk of harbouring scalp metastases, for example those with leukaemia or multiple myeloma, since the vasoconstrictive effect will prevent cytotoxics from reaching the tumour cells as well as the hair follicles.

Many centres do not use tourniquets or scalp cooling but simply explain to the patient that alopecia may occur, stressing that the hair will grow again on completion of chemotherapy (and sometimes during treatment). It is also made clear that the hospital will provide a wig, matching the patient's present style and colouring, during the period of alopecia. With these assurances hair loss during chemotherapy is usually accepted by most patients.

Drug Extravasation

A number of cytotoxic drugs cause intense local inflammation, resulting in pain and sometimes progressing to necrosis and ulceration, if they leak from the vein during administration. Ideally good injection technique should avoid this complication but even when the greatest care and skill are exercised such accidents still occasionally occur.

If extravasation is suspected then the injection must be stopped immediately, pressure on the syringe reversed – to aspirate as much of the drug as possible – and the needle withdrawn. There have been various reports suggesting that local injection of either corticosteroids (to reduce inflammation) or sodium bicarbonate (to neutralise the acidity of most cytotoxic solutions) around the site of leakage may be beneficial, but clear evidence for this is lacking. Elevation of the affected limb together with immediate application of ice packs over the area of extravasation does appear to reduce the risk of tissue necrosis. Elevation should be maintained for 48 hours and ice packs applied for 15 minutes, four times daily.

If, after 48 hours, the reaction has settled then the patient may begin to use the arm normally again, although he should be advised to keep it elevated whenever possible. If there is immediate evidence of ulceration or if pain, erythema, blistering or swelling persist at the injection site after 48 hours, then the opinion of a plastic surgeon should be sought to advise whether early excision and skin grafting is indicated, in order to avoid chronic ulceration.

Antagonism of Cytotoxic Action

There are no universal antidotes available to reverse the side effects of cytotoxic drugs, but two preparations do exist which help reduce the toxicity specific agents: these preparations are leucovorin and mesna.

Leucovorin

Methotrexate acts by inhibiting the enzyme dihydrofolate reductase. This enzyme carries out the reduction of dihydrofolic acid to tetrahydrofolic acid, which is then transformed to a number of tetrahydrofolates, which are essential co-factors for purine and pyrimidine synthesis (see Figure 3.5). This enzyme blockade may be overcome by giving leucovorin (folinic acid). Leucovorin is a tetrahydrofolate and is readily converted to other, closely related, tetrahydrofolates needed to restore nucleic acid synthesis. It has recently been suggested that, in addition to simply circumventing the metabolic block caused by methotrexate, leucovorin might also competitively displace methotrexate from dihydrofolate reductase, allowing reactivation of the enzyme (Figure 5.1). Furthermore there is experimental evidence that this reaction occurs more readily in normal cells than in tumour cells, thus preferentially rescuing normal cells from the harmful effects of methotrexate.

Giving leucovorin after methotrexate administration therefore offers a means of antagonising the cytotoxic activity of the latter drug and preventing

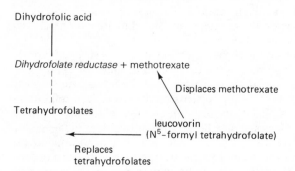

Figure 5.1.   The role of leucovorin in reversing the action of methotrexate (see also Figure 3.5).

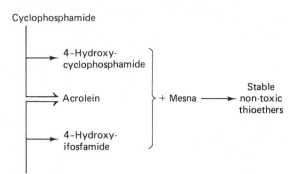

Figure 5.2. The interaction of mesna and urotoxic metabolites of cyclophosphamide and ifosfamide.

further toxicity. This forms the basis of the technique of leucovorin-rescue which allows very high doses of methotrexate to be given and then followed 24 to 36 hours later by leucovorin (given orally or by intramuscular injection) in order to prevent toxicity to resting normal tissue stem cells recruited into the cell cycle following the initial cytotoxic insult.

Leucovorin can only be used to prevent *further* methotrexate toxicity and has no effect on cells already damaged by the drug. In those cases where severe side effects are already apparent appropriate measures will be required to control these, in addition to the administration of leucovorin.

Mesna

Ifosfamide and high doses of cyclophosphamide are both likely to cause haemorrhagic cystitis, and urotoxicity was a dose-limiting factor for ifosfamide in particular until the introduction of mesna. Acrolein and the 4-hydroxy metabolites of these two drugs are thought to be the compounds principally responsible for bladder toxicity (see Chapter 3). Mesna is a sulphydryl-containing agent which reacts with acrolein and the 4-hydroxy metabolites, converting them to other compounds (Figure 5.2) which have no damaging effect on bladder epithelium and so prevents the development of haemorrhagic cystitis. Mesna has no effect on the therapeutic activity of ifosfamide and cyclophosphamide.

Mesna is given intravenously or orally but has a relatively short half-life in the body so care must be taken to see that its administration is continued long enough to ensure complete inactivation of urinary metabolites, particularly in patients with impaired liver or renal function, in whom metabolism and excretion of ifosfamide and cyclophosphamide might be delayed.

Chapter 6
The Safe Handling of Cytotoxic Drugs

Introduction

It is now recognised that cytotoxic drugs represent a health hazard for those
members of hospital staff who are regularly involved in their preparation and
administration. There are two principal risks – one definite and one potential.
The definite risk results from the fact that a number of cytotoxic agents are
extremely irritant and produce harmful local effects after direct contact with
skin or eyes. The potential risk stems from the knowledge that some cytotoxic
drugs are proven carcinogens (see Chapter 2) and a number of studies
monitoring hospital staff who were involved in preparing or giving these
agents have demonstrated chromosomal abnormalities and excretion of
mutagenic products in the urine. The abnormalities disappeared once exposure ceased and the actual amount of drug absorbed was extremely small.
Nevertheless it has been argued that prolonged contact in this way could
increase the chance of later developing a cancer. It is important to stress that
this is only a theoretical possibility and that there is, as yet, no definite link
between previous professional contact with cytotoxics and subsequent development of cancer. Even so, the possibility of a long-term hazard has to be
taken seriously and the Health and Safety Executive in the United Kingdom,
has issued Guidance Notes for the safe handling of cytotoxic drugs and these
have been expanded by many Health Authorities into detailed policy
documents, spelling out the necessary precautions.

Cytotoxic drugs may enter the body by three possible routes: inhalation
(when an aerosol or airborne dust is produced), ingestion or skin contact.
These are most likely to occur with injectable agents during either their
preparation or administration. The rest of this chapter offers guidance on the
general precautions necessary during these procedures.

Precautions During the Preparation of Injectable Cytotoxic Drugs

In any unit where the number of cytotoxic injections prepared exceeds 10 per day, or 40 per week, preparation should be centralised, usually in the pharmacy under the direction of a pharmacist. Where such a centralised reconstitution service is offered there should be a designated aseptic work station, with a wash hand basin and a bench type vertical downflow laminar air cabinet for the actual handling of the drugs (horizontal laminar flow cabinets are not suitable as they offer no protection for the operator). Apart from increasing safety the adoption of centralised reconstitution does have economic advantages in that it reduces the amount of drug wastage: one estimate has suggested that the amount of drug discarded in a major cancer centre fell from 16 per cent to less than 1 per cent following the introduction of centralised dispensing (Bennett S, British Medical Journal, 288: 194, 1984).

For smaller departments, where centralised dispensing is not appropriate, cytotoxic preparation should be carried out in a specially designated area, such as a side room off a ward or clinic. This should be equipped with a suitable laminate or stainless-steel work surface, with lips or trays to contain spillage. A sink with running water should be available. The windows and doors should be closed to provide a contained environment and the room should not be used for other purposes whilst the preparation is under way.

Although adequate facilities for drug preparation are essential the key to reducing the risk of exposure is good technique and the following points give some advice on this:

1. Work over a suitable container to prevent the spread of any spillage.

2. Prevent high pressure being generated inside sealed vials – when fluids are introduced an equivalent volume of air should be withdrawn or a venting needle with a hydrophobic filter (to prevent aerosol formation) may be used.

3. Ampoules should be directed away from the face and covered with a suitable pad when broken open.

4. Diluent fluid should be introduced slowly into open ended ampoules or vials, running it down the vessel wall and ensuring the drug powder is moist before shaking.

5. When excess air is expelled from a filled syringe it should be exhausted into a pad and not straight into the atmosphere.

6. If excess drug is to be expelled from the syringe the needle should be removed first and sterile cotton wool placed over the end of the syringe to prevent possible scatter of aerosol droplets.

7. Luer lock fittings should be used in preference to push connections on syringes, tubing and giving sets.

Precautions for Administration of Cytotoxic Drugs

The training and observance of good technique, as outlined above, is essential. Personal protective clothing is also advisable, as follows:

1. Skin protection: suitable gloves are needed. Usually PVC disposable gloves are adequate (although latex gloves are needed for amsacrine) and disposable plastic gowns or aprons are advised.

2. Eye protection: protective eye goggles or industrial spectacles with plastic sidepieces.

3. Surgical face mask: to prevent inhalation of drug.

If any spillage occurs this should be dealt with as soon as possible by the staff member who has administered the drug (mopping up must not be delegated to the domestic staff). The spilt material should be mopped up with disposable absorbent towels which should then be double bagged and sent for incineration. Contaminated surfaces should be washed with copious volumes of water. Gloves used during mopping up should be disposed of in the same way as other contaminated solid waste (see below) and fresh gloves should be put on before continuing with other work.

Following drug administration all sharps should be placed in an impenetrable container specified for the purpose and sent for incineration. All other solid disposable equipment (syringes, drug containers, gloves, cotton wool, aprons, face masks) should be double bagged, marked with a "Biohazard" label and sent for incineration. Non-disposable items, such as goggles, should be washed with large volumes of water whilst the operator is wearing protective gloves and an apron.

These guidelines offer some general principles for the safe handling of injectable cytotoxic drugs and Table 6.1 gives specific advice for individual agents. Although the risk of contamination is greatest with injectable preparations there is a theoretical danger of absorption from excessive handling of tablets or capsules and those staff with regular and prolonged exposure to these preparations should ensure they always wear disposable gloves when handling them.

Table 6.1.   Guidelines for the preparation and administration of injectable cytotoxic drugs

Drug presentation and storage	Reconstitution, administration	Special comments
Actinomycin-D: 500mcg vials. Refrigerate	Add 1.1ml water for injection. For iv bolus injection add a further 9ml water for injection and either give slowly directly into vein or into tubing of fast-running drip. For iv infusion add dose to 5% dextrose solution or normal saline	Very corrosive so avoid extravasation. Solution must be freshly prepared, discard any unused solution. Some drug may be removed by cellulose ester membrane filters
Amsacrine: 75mg in 1.5ml ampoule plus diluent	Add each ampoule to 13.5ml of lactic acid diluent to give a solution of 5mg per ml of the drug. Add required dose to 500ml 5% dextrose and infuse over 60 to 90 minutes	Use glass syringes as leaching of substances from the plunger of plastic syringes may occur. Irritant to skin and soft tissues: avoid skin contact and extravasation, use latex gloves (not PVC)
Asparaginase: 10,000 unit vials. Refrigerate	Add 1–2ml normal saline or water for injection to each vial, shake gently. Give by im or sc route. For slow iv bolus injection add further 9ml normal saline. For iv infusion add to normal saline and give by rapid infusion over 20–30 min	Give test dose of 50 units intradermally to exclude hypersensitivity, if reaction appears within 3 hr do not give drug. Prepared solution to be used within 24 hr for iv bolus or 12 hr for infusions
Bleomycin: 5mg and 15mg ampoules. May be stored at room temperature	For im use add up to 5ml of normal saline to 15mg amp. For iv use add 5ml saline to 15mg amp and give as bolus injection over 1–2 min or add to further normal saline for infusion. For intracavitary injection add required dose to 100ml saline	Avoid skin contact and extravasation. The im injection may cause local pain; 2ml 1% lignocaine used as solvent to avoid discomfort. Solution must be freshly prepared
Carboplatin: 150mg vials. Refrigerate	Add 15ml water for injection to each vial then dilute with normal saline or 5% dextrose for infusion over 15–60 min	Solutions should be used within 8 hr
Carmustine: 100mg vials. Refrigerate: If drug appears as oily film at bottom of vial this indicates decomposition and the vial should be discarded	Add 3ml alcohol diluent to each vial then add 27ml water for injection. The required dose is added to 5% dextrose or normal saline for infusion over 1–2 hr	Avoid skin contact and extravasation. Bolus injection and rapid infusion under one hour may cause great pain at injection site. Solutions are stable for 2 hr at room temperature and 20 hr at 4°C

Table 6.1 (*continued*)

Drug presentation and storage	Reconstitution, administration	Special comments
Cisplatin: 10mg and 50mg vials containing powder for reconstitution, also vials of 10mg in 20ml or 50mg in 100ml as prepared solution. Refrigerate	Reconstitute powder with 10ml water for injection for 10mg vials. Add appropriate dose of reconstituted solution or prepared solution to either normal saline or dextrose–saline and infuse either rapidly or up to 20 hr	Establish iv hydration before giving drug and for 24 hr afterwards to reduce risk of renal damage. Use reconstituted powder and infusions within 24 hr, protect from strong sunlight and do not refrigerate as precipitation occurs
Cyclophosphamide: 100mg, 200mg, 500mg and 1g vials. Store in a cool place	To 100mg vial add 5ml, to 200mg vial add 10ml, to 500mg vial add 25ml and to 1g vial add 50ml of water for injection. Give by bolus injection over 1–2 min. For high-dose therapy add 500ml dextrose-saline and infuse over 1–2 hr	Slow to dissolve. Solution must be freshly prepared and used within 8 hr. When doses exceed 1g per m^2 mesna should be given to prevent haemorrhagic cystitis
Cytosine arabinoside: 100mg vials with diluent or 2ml and 5ml ampoules containing 40 and 100mg of drug, respectively, in prepared solution. Refrigerate but do not freeze	To 100mg vial add 5ml of the diluent provided for iv use or 1ml for subcutaneous injection. Solutions may be given iv by bolus injection over 1–2 min or, with the addition of normal saline or 5% dextrose, by infusion over up to 24 hr. If drug is to be given intrathecally use saline for reconstitution of powder and not the diluent	Solutions should be freshly made and used within 48 hr; if solution becomes hazy it should be discarded
Dacarbazine: 100mg and 200mg vials. Refrigerate	To 100mg vial add 9.9ml, to 200mg vial add 19.7ml of water for injection. Concentrated solutions are painful when injected so either dilute to 50ml and give by bolus injection over 1–2 min or add required dose to 200ml 5% dextrose or normal saline and infuse over 30 min	Avoid contact with skin and eyes. Avoid extravasation. The reconstituted solution is photosensitive so protect from light. Solution should be freshly prepared and is stable for 8hr at room temperature or 72hr at 4°C
Daunorubicin: 20mg vials. May be stored at room temperature	To 20mg vial add 5ml normal saline then either make up required dose to 20ml with saline and inject via tubing of fast running saline drip over 3–5 min or give as infusion in 100ml saline	Avoid extravasation and flush through well after administration. Freshly prepared solutions may be stored away from light for up to 48hr

(*continued next page*)

Table 6.1 (*continued*)

Drug presentation and storage	Reconstitution, administration	Special comments
Doxorubicin: 10mg and 50mg vials. May be stored at room temperature	To 10mg vial add 5ml, to 50mg vial add 25ml water for injection. Either inject into tubing of fast running saline drip over 3–5 min or give as slow bolus injection in 50ml water or saline with great care or as 50–100ml infusion in saline. For instillation into the bladder dissolve 50mg of drug in 50ml normal saline; the solution is retained in the bladder for 60 min	Avoid extravasation and flush through well after administration. Freshly prepared solutions may be stored for 24 hr at room temperature or 48 hr at 4°C
Epirubicin: 10mg, 20mg and 50mg vials. May be stored at room temperature	To 10mg vial add 5ml, to 20mg vial add 10ml and to 50mg add 25ml water for injection. Then inject in tubing of fast running saline drip or give in minibag of 50–100ml normal saline	Use freshly prepared solution within 24 hr
Etoposide: 100mg ampoules. Store below 40°C	Ampoules contain 100mg of drug in 5ml. Dilute required dose with normal saline to a concentration of 0.25mg/ml or less (higher concentrations may cause precipitation) and give by iv infusion over at least 30 min	Avoid skin contact and extravasation. Very rapid infusion may cause hypotension; anaphylactic reactions have been seen. Use freshly prepared solution within 6hr
5-Fluorouracil: 250mg in 10ml, in ampoules and 500mg in 20ml in vials. Store between 10° and 30°C. Protect from light	Solutions may be given by slow iv bolus injection or may be added to 500ml normal saline or 5% dextrose and infused over 4 hr	Avoid extravasation. Infusions solutions should be used within 24 hr and protected from light
Ifosfamide: 500mg, 1g and 2g vials. May be stored at room temperature	Reconstitute powder with 6.5ml water for 500mg vial, 12.5ml for 1g and 25ml for 2g. For iv bolus use dilute with an equal volume of water. For infusion add required dose to dextrose saline or normal saline and give over 30–120 min or make up in 3l and infuse over 24 hr	Use freshly prepared solution. Ensure adequate hydration and give mesna to prevent haemorrhagic cystitis
Melphalan: 100mg vials with solvent and diluent. May be stored at room temperature	Mix 1ml of solvent with 100mg, shake at once, then add 9ml of diluent. Inject required dose into tubing of fast running normal saline drip or give by saline infusion in 8 hr or less	Avoid extravasation. Unstable in dextrose solutions. Stable in saline for up to 8 hr. Use freshly prepared solution

Table 6.1 (*continued*)

Drug presentation and storage	Reconstitution, administration	Special comments
Methotrexate: 2.5mg, 5mg, 25mg, 50mg or 250mg vials of drug in isotonic solution. 50mg, 500mg, 1g or 5g vials with drug as powder. May be stored at room temperature	Powder in the 50mg vial is reconstituted with 2ml water and contains parabens as preservative. Powder in 500mg, 1g and 5g vials requires water for reconstitution but has no preservatives. Solutions may be given by direct iv injection or by infusion when added to normal saline or 5% dextrose	Only preservative-free solutions should be used for intrathecal and intravenous routes. Solutions should be freshly prepared and used within 24 hr, infusions should be protected from bright sunlight
Mithramycin: 2.5mg vials. Refrigerate	Add 4.9ml water for injection and shake to dissolve. Add required dose to 1l 5% dextrose and infuse over 4 to 6 hr	Avoid extravasation. Avoid iv bolus injection as it leads to increased risk of gastrointestinal side effects. Use freshly prepared solution
Mitomycin-C: 2mg, 10mg and 20mg vials May be stored at room temperature	To 2mg vial add 5ml, to 10mg add at least 10ml and to 20mg add at least 20ml water for injection. Give by slow iv bolus injection over 1–2 min or add to 500ml 5% dextrose and infuse over 1hr. For bladder instillation the required dose should be dissolved in 20–40ml water	Avoid extravasation. Solutions should be freshly prepared and protected from light
Mitozantrone: 20mg, 25mg and 30mg vials as 2mg per ml solution	Dilute contents of vial(s) to at least 50ml with 5% dextrose, normal saline or dextrose saline and give through tubing of iv infusion over 3 min, or add to 100ml normal saline and infuse over 15–30 min	Solutions stable in glass or plastic for 24hr. Do not freeze
Nitrogen mustard: 10mg vials. Refrigerate	Add 10ml normal saline to each vial. Inject required dose into tubing of fast running saline or 5% dextrose drip over 2 min	Avoid extravasation and skin contact – very corrosive. Solutions must be freshly prepared and used within 30 min
Thiotepa: 15mg vials	To 15mg vial add 1.5ml water for injection. For bladder instillation prepare 30–60mg of drug in 60ml water. For intra-cavity use add 20ml water for each 15mg vial. May also be given by direct iv bolus injection	If precipitate forms on adding water polymerisation has occurred and drug should be discarded. Solutions chemically stable for 5 days but as they have no preservative discard after 24 hr

(*continued next page*)

Table 6.1 (*continued*)

Drug presentation and storage	Reconstitution, administration	Special comments
Vinblastine: 10mg vials with 10ml diluent. Refrigerate	Add 10ml of water for injection or diluent provided. Give by iv bolus injection over 1 min or into tubing of fast running 5% dextrose or normal saline infusion	Avoid extravasation. Solutions reconstituted with water may be kept refrigerated for 48hr, solutions reconstituted with diluent may be kept refrigerated for 30 days
Vincristine: 1mg and 2mg vials of drug in solution. 1mg, 2mg and 5mg vials with diluent. Refrigerate	To 1mg or 5mg vial add 10ml diluent provided or water for injection or normal saline. Inject directly into vein over 1 min or into tubing of running saline infusion	Avoid extravasation. If diluent used, solution may be stored in refrigerator for 14 days; for other solutions use within 24 hr
Vindesine: 5mg vials with diluent. Refrigerate	To 5mg vial add 5ml diluent provided or 5ml normal saline. Give by direct injection into vein over 1–3 min or into tubing of running saline or 5% dextrose infusion	Avoid extravasation. If diluent used solution may be stored in refrigerator for 30 days, if saline may be kept in refrigerator for 48hr

Chapter 7

Resistance to Cytotoxic Drugs

Introduction

Tumour resistance to cytotoxic therapy may be primary or secondary. Tumours which show no response to drug administration are said to be primarily resistant. In other cancers regression is seen initially but in many cases the benefit is only temporary and, after a variable period of time, the tumour will reappear and the patient relapse despite continuing chemotherapy. This progression of disease during treatment indicates that the tumour has developed secondary resistance to the particular drugs being given. A change of agents at this time may well bring about a further remission.

Cytotoxic drug resistance may be due to a number of general factors which operate before the drug reaches the cancer cell and may result in apparent resistance even when the cancer cells themselves are sensitive to the given agent. Alternatively resistance may be due to specific features of the tumour cell which enable it to survive.

General Factors

Timing of Drug Administration

It is quite possible for a cancer to be sensitive to a particular drug but to fail to show any clinical response simply because the scheduling of drug administration is incorrect. As we saw in Chapter 4, this could occur simply because the interval between courses of cytotoxic therapy is too long, enabling the tumour to increase in size between treatments even though it is sensitive to the drug that is being given. It is not yet possible to study the kinetics of tumours in every patient and plan treatment schedules accordingly, so the frequency of failure due to excessive gaps between treatments is uncertain.

A more specific area where drug scheduling may affect clinical outcome is the administration of cell-cycle phase-specific agents. These have their maximal effect on tumour cells at certain times during the cell cycle. If the drug has a relatively short half-life in the body and is given by intermittent bolus injections then only a relatively small proportion of cells will be exposed to the drug during their sensitive phase. If the drug is given by continuous infusion over several days then a far greater percentage of the cancer cells will move into the sensitive phase during that time, with a proportional increase in cell kill. Cytosine arabinoside is a phase-specific drug with a plasma half-life of only a few hours and both laboratory and clinical studies have clearly shown the importance of scheduling for this agent (Table 7.1).

Table 7.1. The influence of dose scheduling on the efficacy of cytosine arabinoside in acute myeloid leukaemia. (Freireich. E et al. (1969) Cancer Research. **27**: 573–577)

Dose	Response rate	
	Complete	Partial
Daily iv bolus injections on 5 consecutive days	12.5%	0
Continuous iv infusion for 5 consecutive days	43%	15%

Anatomical Isolation

During the 1960s combination chemotherapy achieved dramatic results in the treatment of acute lymphatic leukaemia in children. Subsequent follow-up, however, showed a high proportion of patients relapsing eighteen months to two years after their initial treatment with leukaemic infiltration of the central nervous system, previously considered to be a rare complication. The relapses occurred because none of the drugs being used at that time were able to cross the blood-brain barrier. This meant that microscopic leukaemic deposits in the brain and spinal cord were able to grow undisturbed. The addition of CNS irradiation or intrathecal methotrexate to treatment protocols has now overcome this complication.

Failure to penetrate the blood–brain barrier is a special example of anatomical isolation of tumours from drug action. A much commoner form of anatomical isolation occurs in many solid tumours where cytotoxics fail to reach the anoxic centres of the tumour mass because of the poor blood supply. Viable tumour cells are often present in these anoxic regions and will survive to repopulate the growth after treatment, thereby causing a relapse.

In both these examples the drug resistance is apparent rather than real and simply reflects a failure of the cytotoxic agent to reach tumour cells which might well be susceptible to attack.

Drug Antagonism

In laboratory experiments a number of interactions between cytotoxic drugs have been observed in which two agents which are normally active produce a reduced tumour cell kill when they are given together. The two best documented examples of this antagonism of antitumour effect both involve methotrexate. In the one, methotrexate is inhibited by pretreatment with asparaginase; in the other it is inhibited by pretreatment with 5-fluorouracil (although giving 5-fluorouracil after methotrexate leads to potentiation of activity). Various biochemical explanations have been put forward to explain these observations. No clear evidence has emerged from clinical studies to indicate that scheduling of these drugs is important. For the present the possibility of apparent drug resistance due to antagonism remains a theoretical concept rather than a clinical reality.

Antibody Formation

One mechanism of resistance that has been definitely established for asparaginase is the development by the patient of neutralising antibodies which render the drug ineffective.

Cellular Factors Causing Drug Resistance

Two theories have been put forward to account for the development of cellular drug resistance. The first suggests that the tumour population is far from uniform and is made up of many varied families, or clones, of cells, each with slightly different biological properties, and that among this heterogeneous population a number of cells will have inherent drug resistance to the action of a given cytotoxic drug. As treatment continues the sensitive cells will be destroyed but the primarily resistant population will not be affected and will expand to repopulate the tumour; so after an initial period of regression tumour growth will continue as before. The second theory suggests that the resistance is acquired as a result of the appearance, during treatment, of mutant tumour cells which are unaffected by the given cytotoxic drug. By a process of natural selection these resistant cells will then proliferate and come to dominate the tumour population.

These two theories can be incorporated into a single hypothetical model. Cancers are thought to originate as a result of cellular mutations which allow an individual cell, or group of cells, to escape from normal control mechanisms. In such an unstable population further mutations are likely to occur with the passage of time and some of these mutant cells may carry structural or biochemical abnormalities which render them resistant to cytotoxic agents. This would result in a subpopulation of clones of inherently resistant cells. Many cytotoxic drugs are themselves mutagenic agents and when drug treatment begins the rate of mutation may be expected to increase with the appearance of further resistant clones.

As well as explaining the development of cellular drug resistance this model also offers an additional reason for the generally greater sensitivity of more rapidly dividing tumours to cytotoxic agents, as the more rapidly growing the tumour the shorter its overall lifespan and the less time there has been for resistant mutants to appear. Similarly, if this model is a true representation of events, it provides a further argument for adjuvant therapy, in that the earlier cytotoxic treatment is given the less chance there is of resistant strains having emerged.

A number of suggestions have been put forward to account for the actual mechanisms of cellular drug resistance. Most of these have been demonstrated in animal or tissue culture models but few have so far been proven in man. The following are some of the mechanisms that have been proposed.

Alterations to the Cell Membrane

In order to reach their nuclear target cytotoxic drugs must cross the cell membrane. For a number of drugs this process occurs by passive diffusion but for others active transport mechanisms exist and failure of these means that the drug will not be able to enter the cell. Impaired membrane transport into the cell has been implicated as a cause of resistance to methotrexate and the alkylating agents. Recently much attention has focussed on a different aspect of membrane function: removal of drug from the cell. Studies have shown that some tumour cells develop multiple drug resistance to a group of agents which normally enter the cell by passive diffusion: these are doxorubicin, daunorubicin, actinomycin-D, mithramycin, etoposide, teniposide and the vinca alkaloids. There is now good evidence that this particular form of resistance is due to specific genetic changes which result in an active efflux mechanism which allows the membrane actually to remove these drugs from the cells, thereby reducing their intracellular concentration and diminishing their cytotoxicity.

Increased Drug Deactivation

Tumour cells may develop modified enzyme systems to destroy the drug when it enters the cell and before it can reach the nucleus. This has been observed as one form of resistance to methotrexate.

Loss of Drug Activation Process

Many cytotoxics require intracellular modification before they become active and resistance may occur if the necessary activating enzymes are lost. One of the best documented examples of this is 6-mercaptopurine resistance. This agent requires intracellular conversion to thioinosinic acid in order to be cytotoxic. This conversion is mediated by the enzyme hypoxanthineguanine-phosphoribosyltransferase and it has been observed that this enzyme has been lost in cells which have become resistant to 6-mercaptopurine. Decreased activity of the same enzyme also accounts for resistance to 6-thioguanine (and explains why the two agents are cross resistant). Cytosine arabinoside is activated by the enzyme deoxycytidine kinase and a spectrum of enzymes is needed for the conversion of 5-fluorouracil to its active form. For both these agents decreased enzyme activity is one cause of drug resistance.

Increased Production of Target Molecule

The best known example of this form of resistance is seen with methotrexate therapy. Methotrexate acts by combining with the enzyme dihydrofolate reductase thereby inhibiting the conversion of folic acid to tetrahydrofolates. It has been demonstrated, both in animals and man, that resistance to methotrexate may develop as the result of excessive production of dihydrofolate reductase by the tumour cells so that there is sufficient enzyme to bind with all the methotrexate and still leave some free enzyme to maintain normal metabolism.

Change in Enzyme Specificity

The target enzyme for a given cytotoxic antimetabolite may be modified within the cell so that it is able to distinguish between the false metabolite and the true compound needed for nuclear protein synthesis, so preventing the formation of irreversible enzyme-cytotoxic complexes. This is a second mechanism of resistance to 6-mercaptopurine.

Production of Non-essential Competitors

The cell may produce large amounts of a non-essential compound which has the ability to combine with the cytotoxic rendering it inactive before it reaches its nuclear target. This has been reported in some animal systems following treatment with alkylating agents.

Alternative Biochemical Pathways

Some cytotoxics act by binding irreversibly to an essential enzyme, but the cell may subsequently become resistant to that drug by developing an alternative biochemical pathway for protein or nucleic acid synthesis which no longer requires the original target enzyme. This is one of the ways in which resistance to 5-fluorouracil develops.

Repair of Cytotoxic Damage

Following treatment with alkylating agents it has been reported that some cells develop the ability to excise those sections of the DNA chain affected by cross-linkages, caused by alkylation, and repair the damaged area. Repair mechanisms have also been noted in methotrexate resistance, where cells develop the ability to split the normally irreversible complex formed between methotrexate and dihydrofolate reductase.

Table 7.2. Summary of intracellular drug resistance

Drug	Impaired membrane transport into cell	Development of active efflux mechanism to remove drug from cell	Increased drug deactivation	Loss of drug activation process	Increased production of target molecule	Change in enzyme specificity	Production of non-essential competitors	Development of alternative biochemical pathway	Repair of cytotoxic damage
Alkylating agents	+						+		+
Methotrexate	+		+		+				+
5-Fluorouracil				+				+	
Cytosine arabinoside				+					
6-Mercaptopurine				+		+			
6-Thioguanine				+					
Vinca alkaloids		+							
Anthracyclines		+							
Actinomycin-D		+							
Mithramycin		+							
Etoposide		+							
Teniposide		+							

Prevention of Drug Resistance

At present our ability to predict and avoid the development of drug resistance in individual tumours is very limited. In theory two general principles which should help minimise the development of resistance are to treat the cancer as rapidly as possible and to do so with a combination of cytotoxic drugs.

Rapid treatment means treating the cancer as early as possible in its lifespan when the number of resistant clones will be at a minimum. It also means giving effective chemotherapy over as short a time as possible so that the opportunity for drug resistance to develop during treatment is also minimised.

Combining several drugs with different anticancer actions in a single treatment regime is of value since cells which are resistant to one agent may well be sensitive to another. A recent logical extension of this concept is the suggestion that for those cancers where the number of active drugs is greater than can be accommodated in a single combination, alternating cycles of treatment are given with two different combinations of non-cross-resistant drugs. This approach is showing promising results in the treatment of lymphomas though it has so far been disappointing in solid tumours.

At a cellular level, recent laboratory studies have shown that the cell membrane changes leading to multiple drug resistance may be reversed by a variety of non-cytotoxic drugs. These agents include cyclosporin-A, verapamil, reserpine and tamoxifen. Whether these observations can be exploited clinically to reverse or prevent drug resistance remains to be seen.

Cross Resistance

When choosing a treatment regime for patients who have relapsed on cytotoxic chemotherapy it is important to avoid including drugs which are cross resistant with other agents that have been given previously. The extent to which different cytotoxics are cross resistant is still largely unclear. In the past one widely used guideline was to select agents with differing modes of action: thus a patient who relapsed during treatment with an alkylating agent would receive an antimetabolite or antibiotic rather than a second alkylating agent. This approach may well be unduly restrictive. For example there is evidence that if resistance to alkylating agents occurs due to changes in membrane transport then all members of the group are affected, but if other mechanisms are involved (repair of damage, increased deactivation) then only specific drugs are inhibited and other alkylating agents will still be effective. The development of multiple drug resistance due to membrane changes has now been well established in a number of laboratory studies, but the extent to which it is relevant in man remains to be clarified. One of the few examples of cross resistance to be confirmed in patients is between 6-mercaptopurine and 6-thioguanine, where development of resistance to the one drug is almost invariably accompanied by the appearance of resistance to the other.

Chapter 8

Alternative Methods of Cytotoxic Drug Administration

Introduction

Cytotoxic drugs are usually given by bolus injection, or infusion, into a peripheral vein, or orally as tablets or capsules. Over the years a number of other methods of administration have been devised to try and ensure optimal drug delivery in a variety of different clinical situations. This chapter summarises these techniques, their rationale and indications.

Central Venous Access

Peripheral veins become thrombosed with repeated injections and infusions of cytotoxics: this process is exacerbated in those patients requiring multiple blood tests and infusions of other agents such as blood products, nutrients and antibiotics. In addition the multiple venepunctures involved in these procedures become very distressing for patients who are often extremely ill. Working with leukaemic patients undergoing bone marrow transplantation Hickman and his colleagues in Seattle developed an alternative approach (Hickman RO et al., Surgery Gynecology & Obstetrics, 148: 871–875, 1979). They devised a catheter, which has subsequently become known as a Hickman line, for insertion into the superior vena cava, which could remain in place for weeks or months and provide a single route for withdrawal of blood samples and infusion of cytotoxics, nutritional supplements, blood products and other agents.

The catheter is made of silicone rubber (Silastic) and has an internal diameter of 0.32mm (sufficient to allow withdrawal of blood samples or infusion of nutrients with the minimum risk of blockage). It is in two parts – a thinner intravascular part and a thicker extravascular portion. Two polyester fibre (Dacron) cuffs help to keep the catheter in position at the points of entry into the vein and skin respectively. The catheter is inserted under either local or general anaesthetic. An incision is made over the right or left cephalic vein and forceps are then used to make a subcutaneous tunnel to a point at the level of the fourth or fifth intercostal space, adjacent to the sternum. A further incision is made at this point and the catheter is inserted. It is passed through the subcutaneous passage and into the vein. Under radiologic control it is then advanced until the tip of the catheter comes to lie at the lower end of the superior vena cava where it enters the right atrium. The catheter is then secured by sutures (Figure 8.1). A subsequent modification has been the introduction of double lumen catheters, so that incompatible drugs or solutions may be infused simultaneously.

This technique has obvious advantages for patients in whom repeated venous access is necessary and for those whose peripheral veins have become too thrombosed for further use. It has also allowed the development of continuous ambulatory infusion techniques (see Chapter 4) and a variety of portable pumps are now available for attachment to the catheter in order to provide a constant supply of drug. The routine of catheter care is simple and easily learnt by the patient: it consists of a daily aseptic dressing and flushing the catheter with heparin after use. When the catheter is not in use heparin is left in the tube and is replaced once daily.

The main complications of the Hickman line are haemorrhage in the post-operative period (which is commoner in thrombocytopenic patients), occlusion, which usually requires replacement of the catheter, and infection. Infections may take the form of soft tissue infection of the subcutaneous tunnel or the far more serious complication of bacteraemia and septicaemia. The latter is much more likely in severely leucopenic patients and antibiotic cover is usually given in such cases. These various complications are usually easily managed and do not limit the application of this extremely useful technique.

Intra-arterial Therapy

When a cytotoxic drug is given intravenously it is transported to the heart and thence to the arterial circulation, eventually reaching the tumour via the local arterial blood supply. Thus in order to gain access to the tumour the drug has to be distributed throughout the circulation. Clearly if an equivalent dose of drug was injected directly into the arterial supply of the tumour then a far higher concentration of cytotoxic would be achieved within the lesion, with an equivalent blood level to that seen with intravenous therapy subsequently appearing in the general circulation. Thus the dose of drug received by the tumour (and hence, in theory, the extent of cell kill) would be greatly increased without any increase in systemic toxicity.

This approach could be further exploited if a cytotoxic existed that was almost completely extracted on its first passage through the tumour and was rapidly inactivated or excreted thereafter, so that it reached only minimal concentrations in the general circulation. This would allow ultra-high doses to

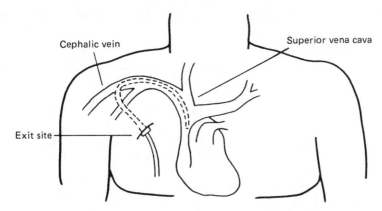

Figure 8.1.   Position of catheter for central venous infusion of cytotoxic drugs.

be given without undue systemic toxicity. Unfortunately none of our existing drugs meet these criteria, so a number of techniques have been devised to try and reduce the risk of systemic side effects. These include giving methotrexate intra-arterially, rapidly followed by intravenous leucovorin in order to inhibit toxicity (see Chapter 5) and the use of pressure cuffs, sometimes combined with intra-arterial balloon catheters, to try and cut off the blood supply *from* the tumour (in order to minimise the amount of drug reaching the rest of the body) or *to* vital organs to protect them from the effects of circulating drug. Another approach is to localise the blood supply of the tumour surgically and employ extracorporeal perfusion to deliver high doses of the drug (see Figure 8.2). This technique is really only applicable for cancers confined to the limbs but has been used with considerable success in soft tissue sarcomas and malignant melanomas of the extremities.

The major disadvantages of intra-arterial therapy are the need for hospital admission and surgery for catheter placement, the complications of having an indwelling arterial catheter (principally haemorrhage, occlusion and infection, as described for intravenous catheters), an increase in toxicity to local tissues around the tumour and the risk of a "geographical miss" of tumour tissue if it derives its blood supply from more than one artery. Intra-arterial chemotherapy was first described in the 1950s and since that time has been used for numerous sites in the body but has only achieved any degree of popularity in four situations: soft tissue sarcomas and melanomas of the limbs, hepatic metastases and head and neck cancer.

Head and Neck Cancer

In the late 1950s and early 1960s infusion of cytotoxics through the carotid arteries was quite extensively evaluated in the management of those patients with squamous cell carcinoma of the head and neck in whom surgery and radiotherapy had nothing more to offer. Methotrexate was the agent of

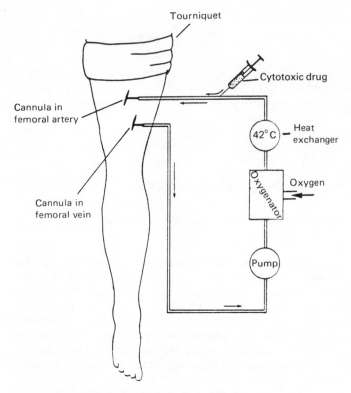

Figure 8.2. Isolated hyperthermic limb perfusion.

choice, having the advantages of proven value against squamous cell carcinoma and rapid neutralisation by leucovorin. A number of series reported
good regressions in advanced disease but the complications were more serious
than in limb perfusion. Mortality directly due to treatment often exceeded 10
per cent with complications such as air embolus, arterial emboli, haemorrhage from the carotid artery, cerebral thrombosis and drug extravasation.
This high mortality and morbidity, combined with improved results from
intermittent intravenous chemotherapy, has now resulted in the virtual
abandonment of regional chemotherapy for advanced head and neck cancer
although it is still occasionally used as an adjuvant to surgery in operable
disease.

Hepatic Metastases

The blood supply of hepatic metastases is almost totally derived from the
hepatic artery and this has led to attempts to treat secondary deposits in the
liver by means of hepatic artery infusions. The group of patients most
frequently treated by this technique are those who have had previous

resections for primary tumours of the large bowel. Catheters can be inserted into the brachial artery, in the arm, and guided, under radiological control, into the hepatic artery. They are then attached to continuous infusion pumps which provide a reservoir of cytotoxic, 5-fluorouracil being the most widely used agent in this indication. Some dramatic results have been claimed in the treatment of hepatic secondaries with this technique but randomised trials are needed to demonstrate a clear superiority, particularly in terms of increased survival, to other treatments. There is, however, some evidence that using this approach as an adjuvant to surgery in patients with large bowel carcinoma may enhance survival. If clinical trials currently in progress confirm a significant improvement in survival then this could become a major indication for intra-arterial chemotherapy.

Malignant Melanoma and Soft Tissue Sarcomas

The majority of malignant melanomas and a significant proportion of soft tissue sarcomas arise from the limbs. Treatment of primary melanomas is wide excision with skin grafting and soft tissue sarcomas are also surgically removed either by amputation or wide excision followed by radiotherapy. Despite these measures local recurrence is not uncommon and only occasionally responds to conventional therapies. In a number of patients isolated limb perfusion with cytotoxics has resulted in considerable benefit. Melphalan has been the drug most widely used although in recent years it has sometimes been combined with actinomycin-D in melanomas and doxorubicin in soft tissue sarcomas. Complications include venous thrombosis, arterial emboli, peripheral nerve damage, local skin reactions and drug extravasation. Despite these problems good results have been seen in many patients with advanced disease. It is now clear that the results may be further improved by combining perfusion with hyperthermia, using an external heat exchanger to raise the temperature of the perfusion fluid to between 40° and 42°C. Hyperthermia is damaging to both oxygenated and hypoxic cells and also increases cytotoxic drug activity and local uptake of cytotoxics. The successes seen with hyperthermic perfusion in advanced disease have resulted in an increasing use of this technique as an adjuvant to initial surgical excision in early disease. Because both these types of cancer are relatively uncommon, prospective controlled trials have not been reported and so absolute confirmation of the value of adjuvant perfusion is still awaited.

A Note on Terminology

Intra-arterial chemotherapy is often referred to as regional chemotherapy since the use of local arteries as the site of injection allows an increase of concentration of the drug in a particular region of the body. In this context the terms infusion and perfusion are often confused. An infusion is the injection of drug into an artery (or vein) with ultimate passage of drug into the general circulation; a perfusion is an attempt to isolate the blood supply of a particular region anatomically, with injection of cytotoxic into the principal artery to that area *together with* its removal by cannulation of the main vein from the area. Thus infusion is simply an injection into the normal circulation, via venous or arterial routes, whilst perfusion involves the establishment of an artifical circulation through the tumour site.

Intrapleural Therapy

Pleural effusions are a frequent complication in a number of common cancers. In men, 50 per cent of effusions occur in patients with lung primaries; lymphomas, leukaemias and gastrointestinal carcinomas account for the bulk of the remaining cases. In women, carcinoma of the breast accounts for some 40 per cent of malignant effusions with ovarian and lung cancers being the other major causes. The presence of an effusion results in dyspnoea and the most rapid way to relieve this is by aspirating the fluid. After aspiration alone more than 60 per cent of effusions will recur. In some cancers systemic therapy will prevent recurrence but it is common practice to instil a small amount of cytotoxic directly into the pleural cavity, through the thoracentesis needle, following complete drainage of the effusion.

In the past alkylating agents, particularly thiotepa and nitrogen mustard, have been used in this situation, but controlled studies have now shown that they prevent recurrence of effusions in fewer than 50 per cent of patients and are little better than aspiration alone. A group of drugs including doxorubicin, bleomycin, quinacrine and tetracycline appear to prevent fluid reaccumulation in 60 to 70 per cent of patients and there is evidence of even higher control rates with *Corynebacterium parvum* and talc, although the latter is associated with very severe local pain which restricts its use. Although a number of controlled trials have now been reported they are all relatively small studies and do not allow definite recommendations for specific agents to be used against individual tumour types. However there is a suggestion that *Corynebacterium parvum* may be more effective in effusions due to lung primaries whereas bleomycin may achieve better control in patients with an underlying breast cancer.

The fact that a number of non-cytotoxic agents appear to have equivalent efficacy to conventional anticancer drugs in this situation suggests that the principal mode of action is one of pleural irritation, with subsequent fibrosis, resulting in a chemical pleurodesis which binds the two layers of the pleura together and so prevents further fluid accumulation, rather than a direct cytotoxic effect on tumour cells.

Systemic toxicity was sometimes seen following instillation of alkylating agents, reflecting their relatively rapid absorption from the pleural cavity which, in turn, probably accounts for their relative lack of efficacy. With the remaining drugs local chest pain for 24 to 48 hours after instillation is the commonest side effect, but this is seldom severe.

Intraperitoneal Therapy

Direct instillation of cytotoxics into the peritoneal cavity has been performed with two different objectives – control of ascites and control of tumour.

Control of Ascites

Secondary deposits of tumour on the peritoneum or omentum lead to the formation of ascites. The development of malignant ascites is an ominous sign, the condition is extremely distressing, the treatment is often inadequate, and it usually heralds the terminal stage of the disease. Temporary relief may be obtained by aspirating the fluid and instilling cytotoxics at the end of the aspiration, in the hope of preventing reaccumulation of fluid. In the past drugs such as thiotepa, nitrogen mustard and cyclophosphamide have been used with only occasional success. More recently bleomycin, doxorubicin and *Corynebacterium parvum* have been given and, although no formal clinical comparisons have been reported, these agents are probably more effective than their predecessors. They are given at the end of aspiration when it is judged that there is still some ascitic fluid remaining to aid in their distribution. After the instillation the patient is asked to roll from side to side to try and achieve the maximum possible distribution of the agent within the peritoneal cavity. Treatment is generally well tolerated but chemical peritonitis is an occasional complication which results in abdominal pain and pyrexia for 24 to 48 hours after instillation.

Control of Tumour

Early attempts at intraperitoneal therapy consisted of either pouring drugs into the peritoneal cavity at the time of initial resection, as a crude form of adjuvant therapy, or giving cytotoxics through a paracentesis needle in the the hope of controlling bulky recurrent intra-abdominal disease: both techniques were essentially unsuccessful. In the last decade better understanding of the pharmacokinetics of intraperitoneal drug administration (largely derived from experience with peritoneal dialysis in renal failure) together with the development of specialised catheters and infusion pumps, allowing continuous drug administration over long periods without the need for repeated abdominal punctures, have resulted in renewed interest in intraperitoneal cytotoxic therapy.

The object of therapy is to maintain the highest possible concentration of drug within the peritoneal cavity for the longest possible time with the minimum of systemic toxicity. In order to achieve these objectives the cytotoxic used should meet the following criteria:

1. The drug should be active against the tumour to be treated.

2. The drug should be capable of killing tumour cells directly without the need for prior activation in other tissues.

3. The drug should be relatively impermeable to the peritoneum so that its systemic absorption is limited.

4. The drug should be rapidly cleared from the plasma.

A number of cytotoxics meet these criteria, including 5-fluorouracil, methotrexate, cisplatinum, mitozantrone, mitomycin-C and doxorubicin. All these agents have been administered intraperitoneally with acceptable toxicity, although dose-limiting abdominal pain was seen with doxorubicin and mitomycin-C at relatively low doses, which probably restricts their use to combination therapy with other drugs rather than as single agents.

Despite the improved time-dose concentrations of drug that may be achieved with the newer delivery systems there is still no evidence of any benefit for patients with peritoneal deposits larger than 1cm in size. This is because the drugs reach the tumour by free-surface diffusion and the degree to which they can penetrate the tumour is very limited. Clinical interest has therefore focussed on adjuvant therapy for the management of patients with tumour nodules of 0.5cm or less in conditions such as ovarian cancer and gastrointestinal carcinoma. The clinical studies carried out to date indicate a possible benefit from treatment but the data are very preliminary and definitive trials are in progress. On the debit side, in addition to potential drug toxicity, problems are frequently encountered with the delivery catheters; these include infection, obstruction of flow, discomfort and hazards such as bowel perforation, bleeding, paralytic ileus and leakage of fluid when the catheter is initially implanted. At present, therefore, intraperitoneal chemotherapy is an active area of research but its place in routine tumour management remains to be defined.

Intravesical Therapy

The majority of bladder carcinomas are first diagnosed at a relatively early stage as superficial, usually papillary, lesions with only limited penetration of the bladder wall. Such tumours are treated by local resection but even when removal appears to be complete recurrences will develop in up to 70 per cent of patients. These often take the form of multiple superficial bladder tumours but in about 10 per cent of patients invasive carcinomas will develop with penetration into the muscular coat of the bladder wall.

Intravesical cytotoxic therapy offers the possibility of a high concentration of the drug being in direct contact with the urothelium for a relatively long time. This has been used both as a direct treatment to try and destroy superficial bladder cancers and also as a prophylactic measure, in an attempt to prevent tumour recurrence after resection. Thiotepa, doxorubicin and mitomycin-C are the principal agents which have been investigated. The drug is instilled through a transurethral catheter and retained for 1 to 2 hours.

Doses and schedules of administration have varied enormously with instillations being repeated weekly or monthly for variable periods of time. These differences in treatment regimes make it difficult to assess the results of therapy. Overall, however, it would seem that when used as active treatment about one third of patients gain complete tumour clearance, one third experience a partial remission and one third show no response. When given prophylactically there is no doubt that the time to recurrence is prolonged and the overall recurrence rate reduced but whether this actually affects the eventual development of *invasive* bladder cancer and enhances survival is still not clear.

Thiotepa, doxorubicin and mitomycin-C all cause local bladder irritation, due to chemical cystitis, in a minority of patients. Thiotepa is well absorbed from the bladder and often gives rise to systemic toxicity. Systemic toxicity is less of a problem with doxorubicin and systemic absorption of mitomycin-C is negligible; as a result the latter two agents continue to be the most actively investigated in intravesical chemotherapy studies.

Intrathecal Therapy

The great majority of cytotoxic drugs are unable to cross the blood–brain barrier. In an attempt to reach tumour deposits within the central nervous system cytotoxic agents have been given by intrathecal injection. This technique has been widely used in the prophylaxis and treatment of CNS deposits in acute leukaemias and lymphomas. Methotrexate has been extensively used in this situation although cytosine arabinoside has also been employed.

Following intravenous infusion of methotrexate the ratio of plasma to cerebrospinal fluid (CSF) concentrations is about 30:1. Therefore intrathecal injection is necessary to achieve cytotoxic levels in the CSF. Usually a maximum dose of 15mg is given and, under normal circumstances, the drug concentration declines in a biphasic pattern with half-lives of 1.7 and 6.6 hours. Clearance may be delayed, however, in patients with raised intracranial pressure, the elderly and those taking probenecid (which inhibits removal of methotrexate from the CSF). Neurotoxicity (see Chapter 3) is probably more likely if clearance of the drug is delayed but the precise relationship between dose/time exposure and the incidence of side effects remains unclear.

Methotrexate is usually administered through a lumbar puncture but it is now clear that when given by this route the concentration of drug achieved in the ventricles of the brain may be only a tenth of that in the spinal canal. To ensure better drug distribution within the CSF Omaya reservoirs (surgically implanted subcutaneous reservoirs connected to a lateral ventricle in the brain) have been used. Infusion of methotrexate through such reservoirs certainly achieves more uniform drug distribution but it is not clear whether clinical results are improved as a result of this approach.

Although very successful in the management of CNS involvement in leukaemias and lymphomas, the use of intrathecal therapy for gliomas and brain secondaries from solid tumours has been uniformly disappointing.

Topical Therapy

A variety of cytotoxics have been incorporated into creams and ointments for the treatment of skin cancer. The most widely used agent is 5 per cent 5-fluorouracil cream which is applied twice daily for up to four weeks. Application often results in local erythema and blistering and the patient is advised to stop the cream if this occurs before the four week course is completed. Because of limited absorption this route of administration is only suitable for extremely superficial lesions and the well established success of surgery and radiotherapy in the treatment of most skin cancers limits the indications for its use. Topical cytotoxic therapy has, however, been shown to give good results in some cases of hyperkeratosis, superficial basal cell carcinomas, carcinoma in situ of the skin (Bowen's disease), erythroplasia of Queyrat (carcinoma in situ of the glans penis) and mycosis fungoides (a form of lymphoma primarily involving the skin).

Chapter 9

The Development and Assessment of New Cytotoxic Drugs

Introduction

In the early days of cancer chemotherapy compounds which showed promising antitumour effects in the laboratory were rapidly given to patients with a minimum of preclinical testing. The subsequent clinical evaluation of toxicity and efficacy was often crude and superficial by today's standards. Stimulated by events such as the thalidomide tragedy, increasing statutory controls on new drug development were introduced during the 1950s and 1960s. During the same period the principles of clinical assessment became more clearly defined and a relatively uniform pattern of evaluation has emerged.

Both in the UK and in the USA new drug development goes through two regulatory phases which broadly equate to preclinical development and clinical evaluation. Successful completion of the preclinical phase results in the granting of a Clinical Trial Certificate (CTC) by the Committee on Safety of Medicines, in the UK and an Investigational New Drug (IND) certificate by the Food and Drugs Administration (FDA) in the USA. Successful completion of clinical testing results in a Product Licence or New Drug Approval (NDA) being granted, in the UK and USA respectively. At this stage the new drug becomes commercially available.

Preclinical Testing

The main components of preclinical evaluation required by the regulatory authorities are manufacturing data and details of preclinical investigations of efficacy and toxicity. The manufacturing data must include information on the following points: the name and chemical structure of the drug, the method for its synthesis and purification, the preparation of the various formulations of the drug and their stability together with a full account of the quality control procedures used at all stages of manufacture in order to guarantee uniformity of purity and potency of the drug.

Preclinical data must show evidence of anticancer activity sufficient to justify clinical evaluation and also results to ensure, as far as possible, that the toxicity of the compound is within acceptable limits. In order to get this information a variety of *in vitro* and *in vivo* screening systems are used.

Every year some 15,000 compounds are submitted to the National Cancer Institute, in the USA, and some 3,000 to the Institut Jules Bordet, in Brussels, for evaluation as possible anticancer agents. In order to handle this number of drugs specific screening systems have been developed including both *in vitro* and *in vivo* tumour models. The *in vitro* systems, although often providing interesting supportive data, are still considered to be too unreliable for definitive testing. Of the *in vivo* models the most widely used have been the transplantable murine tumours and more recently human tumour xenografts grown in immunosuppressed mice. Over the years the mouse leukaemia P388 has become recognised as one of the most sensitive of these tumours and is used by the NCI as a prescreen to monitor for cytotoxic effect. Agents which show activity against this tumour are then tested against a panel of five murine tumours and three human tumour xenografts. These are leukaemia L1210, melanoma B16, colon C6, mammary carcinoma $D8F_1$ and Lewis lung carcinoma with colon CX-2, breast MX-1 and lung LX-1 as the three xenografts. Less than 5 per cent of compounds submitted pass the initial P388 leukaemia screen; of these only a handful each year show sufficient activity in the other tests to justify further development.

If tests with the above systems indicate that a new agent has definite cytotoxic properties then the next stage in the assessment is the study of its pharmacology and its toxic effects. This involves tests in normal animals where the aim is not to monitor the anticancer activity of the drug but to discover such things as its optimum route of administration, stability, metabolism and excretion. Further studies are then performed with different doses and dose schedules to determine the toxicity profile and gain an indication of the maximum tolerated and lethal doses of the new drug. Studies with a variety of experimental animals led to the conclusion that beagle dogs and rhesus monkeys gave the best prediction of qualitative side effects in man and would, if anything, overpredict the degree of toxicity. From these observations the NCI developed a comprehensive programme of preclinical toxicity testing involving dogs, monkeys and mice, but by the end of the 1970s it was realised that the complexity of this protocol was causing unnecessary delays and expense as well as requiring inordinate numbers of experimental animals. From 1980 the system was modified to include simply mouse and dog studies with the option to add testing in rats if this was necessary.

Based on these preclinical investigations the CTC or IND application will include an outline of the planned initial clinical evaluation of the drug and, if approval is given, this will be the next stage of the assessment.

Clinical Evaluation

Over the last twenty years clinical evaluation has developed into a standard pattern which normally goes through three clearly defined phases. The studies involved during each phase are described below:

Phase I Studies

The aims of phase I studies are to assess the maximum tolerated dose of the drug with a given schedule and route of administration and also to define the toxicity profile of the compound. This means not only identifying the side effects which occur but also determining whether they are predictable, tolerable and reversible. No antitumour effect is specifically looked for at this stage, although any responses which do occur are carefully documented in order to give guidance for planning phase II and III trials.

Phase II Studies

Armed with the knowledge of the maximum dose of drug that may be given and its possible hazards in man, the actual anticancer activity of the drug may now be evaluated. Phase II studies involve assessments of efficacy in groups of patients each with a single tumour type. The choice of tumours to be treated depends on indications of response seen in preclinical and Phase I studies. In addition the drug is usually screened against a panel of tumours representing a broad spectrum of malignant disease ranging from slowly growing to very rapidly growing cancers and from those which are rarely sensitive to cytotoxics to those with a high degree of chemosusceptibility. The current panel of tumours recommended by the NCI comprises carcinoma of the colon, breast and bronchus, malignant melanoma, high-grade lymphoma and acute leukaemia.

Traditionally phase II studies have used a single arm design with all patients being given the investigational drug, but more recently a number of experts have advocated randomised phase II evaluations with a control arm in which an established drug, of recognised value in that particular condition, is given. The intention is to give the earliest possible indication of the relative efficacy of the new drug, but such a protocol is clearly only appropriate for those tumours where existing agents have already demonstrated significant activity.

The number of patients to be included in a phase II study depends primarily on the response rate one hopes to see: the less active the drug the greater the number of patients that will be required to demonstrate its activity. This means that the numbers involved are likely to vary with different disease types – for example in breast cancer, where many existing agents show significant antitumour activity, one would require a high response rate from the new agent (or evidence of equivalent response rates with significantly less toxicity than existing drugs) in order to make further evaluation worthwhile, hence relatively few patients would be needed. In tumours such as malignant melanoma and renal cell carcinoma, where results with current agents are generally disappointing, far lower levels of activity would justify further investigation of the new drug and hence larger phase II studies would be needed. Usually the number of patients involved for each tumour type ranges from 15 to 50.

Phase III Studies

If a drug has been shown to have an effect against one or more of the signal tumours, then what remains is for its place in the treatment of that disease to be assessed. This is the aim of phase III clinical studies, where the new drug is tested against existing agents, or other forms of treatment, known to be of value in that condition. The controlled clinical trial forms the cornerstone of phase III testing. In these studies patients are allocated, in a random fashion, either to the new drug under evaluation or a treatment of recognised value for that particular tumour. The results are subsequently analysed and whichever group fares better is deemed to have received the optimum treatment. Such a simple statement hides the many difficulties and potential inaccuracies of such trials and although these studies are the most widely accepted tool for testing new forms of treatment it could be argued, especially in malignant disease, that it is impossible to conduct a totally reliable trial. A detailed discussion of all the pitfalls in the methodology and interpretation of randomised trials is beyond the scope of this book, but a discussion of one key area, the criteria by which the value of a new drug is actually determined, will give an indication of some of the problems that may be encountered.

Criteria of Assessment

A new anticancer drug may prove superior to existing agents in one of two ways: it may be more effective or it may be equally effective but cause substantially less toxicity. Measures of efficacy are based on demonstrating one or more of the following: improved cure rates, improved survival times, improved response rates or improved palliation.

Cure

Perhaps surprisingly, cure remains remarkably difficult to define reliably for cancer patients. Work done in the early part of this century, principally looking at squamous cell carcinoma of the head and neck, suggested that most patients who survived for five years after initial treatment, with no evidence of recurrence, were cured and for many years five-year survival figures were equated with cure. It is now well recognised, however, that for many cancers recurrence may occur as long as ten or even twenty years after primary therapy, and some other measure of cure is therefore necessary.

A patient who experiences complete clinical regression of all cancer following treatment and remains symptom-free until death from other causes would appear to have been cured of the malignancy. Although very satisfactory for the patient this so-called "personal cure" is not an absolute definition as the individual may have been harbouring microscopic metastases at the time of their intercurrent death.

The most widely recognised concept of cure is, therefore, based on statistical considerations and defines a cure as being achieved when the life expectancy of the cancer patient is the same as an individual of the same age and sex in the normal population. This concept of "statistical cure" offers the possibility of determining, from large population studies, the time necessary for the individual to survive, free from relapse, after clinically complete removal or regression of disease, in order to be considered likely to be cured.

Survival

Many trials use duration of survival in order to gauge the success of treatment. This may appear a more finite measure than cure but considerable problems of definition and interpretation may still arise, for example those given below:

Time of Analysis of Survival

In many cancers, especially when dealing with early stage disease, preparing real survival curves, based on times from entry on study until death for all patients in the series, may take many years. Understandably, when evaluating new drugs, such a long delay in assessment is frustrating and so increasing use has been made of statistical methods to predict survival curves before completion of follow-up. One disadvantage of these analyses is that if the group comprises a large number of subjects who have only been included in the study for a short time, and thus have only a limited opportunity for failure on treatment, then the probability of survival is subject to greater variability than with longer follow-up times and may lead to unreliable, usually falsely optimistic, predictions. In order to avoid over-interpretation of such methods it is important to ensure that the *minimum* follow-up time is of sufficient length to include the *majority* of relapses that would be expected in the particular cancer under consideration.

Historical Controls

Another way of reducing the time to evaluation in a trial is to employ historical controls. In this system the results of a new treatment are compared to those seen with a similar group of patients who received a different treatment in the past. This means that one only needs half as many subjects as for a randomised trial, greatly reducing the recruitment period. There is, however, general scepticism about the reliability of historical controls: selection bias, variation in analysis, improvements in ancillary care, better supportive therapy and changes in staging procedures all predispose to a more favourable outcome for the study patients as opposed to their historical counterparts. All too often a new drug has shown a significant advantage in trials using historical controls but has proved to be of no benefit when subsequent randomised studies have been carried out.

Relapse-free Survival

Death is a reasonably well-defined end point (although there may be difficulties with interpretation, for example when a patient dies due to causes other than cancer or when death is directly related to treatment toxicity rather than disease progression). An alternative survival measure is the time from complete disappearance of all tumour until the appearance of local recurrence or distant metastases, the so-called relapse-free survival period. The use of this particular end point is unreliable and may result in confusion. It is unreliable because, whereas death occurs at a specific point in time, identifying the date of relapse is far more difficult and is heavily dependent on how often patients are followed up and how rigorously they are examined and investigated to exclude relapse on each occasion.

The use of relapse-free survival has led to confusion especially in adjuvant studies where there has been a tendency to report relapse-free figures rather than actual survival. This can be particularly misleading in those trials using control arms with no adjuvant therapy. For example, if after apparently curative surgery patients are randomised to receive either no further treatment, or chemotherapy with drugs known to produce complete remission in a significant number of patients with advanced disease, then to compare relapse-free survival for the two groups is giving an advantage to the chemotherapy arm: the patients in the control group who relapse may well go on to have a subsequent complete remission from chemotherapy and so have an equivalent overall survival to a patient who relapsed later but had received chemotherapy initially. There is no doubt that a number of the apparent positive benefits of adjuvant cytotoxic therapy have been due to reliance on relapse-free survival data and that these benefits often disappear when actual survival figures are examined.

Survival by Response

This form of assessment is particularly common in single arm studies of new drugs. In most such series some patients will respond to therapy and others will not: the survival time of the responders is then compared to that of the non-responders. If the responders live longer then this is offered as evidence that treatment improves survival. This may well represent an over-interpretation of the results. It could simply be that those patients who responded possessed certain characteristics in the biology or natural history of their tumours that would have resulted in longer survival even if no treatment had been given; the response (measured in terms of tumour shrinkage) seen with treatment was simply a marker identifying this favoured group, but not influencing the time scale of their disease. Alternatively the survival of non-responders might actually be reduced by the treatment, due to factors such as toxicity.

Response

Over the years response to treatment and reduction in tumour size have tended to become equated in the literature, with measurable tumour shrinkage being the major criterion of successful chemotherapy. Many of the early papers evaluating cytotoxic drugs made little or no attempt to define criteria of response and when such criteria were identified they often varied enormously in different studies, making comparison of the results quite impossible. Since the 1960s there has been increasing adoption of standard definitions of response which may be summarised as: complete response (disappearance of all evidence of tumour); partial response (a greater than 50 per cent reduction in tumour size); minimal response (25 to 50 per cent reduction in size); stable disease (an increase or decrease in tumour size of less than 25 per cent); progressive disease (greater than 25 per cent increase in size). Even so there are still difficulties with these criteria as the following examples show.

Complete Response

This requires complete disappearance of all measurable tumour, but how complete is complete? For example, in assessing the response of an ovarian carcinoma after chemotherapy possible measures might be clinical (disappearance of a previously palpable pelvic mass), radiological (resolution of tumour shown by serial computerised tomography) or pathological (with second-look laparotomy and multiple biopsies confirming clearance of disease). It is likely that a clinical response would be achieved far more frequently than pathological clearance and response rates would be influenced accordingly.

Partial Response

There is almost universal agreement that a partial response represents a greater than 50 per cent reduction in tumour size but how that reduction is measured varies considerably in different series. For example, some trials look for a 50 per cent reduction in diameter of marker lesions, others a 50 per cent reduction in area or the product of two diameters at right angles and others a 50 per cent change in volume. A 50 per cent reduction in diameter, however, represents a far greater degree of tumour shrinkage than a 50 per cent reduction in area or volume. Criteria also vary as to the number of lesions that must show a response. Some protocols specify that all measurable lesions must show a greater than 50 per cent regression, whereas others require only that at least one lesion shows regression, provided that there is no increase in the size of other lesions. Equally there is no general agreement on the time that a response must last in order for it to be considered worthwhile: many studies specify no minimum response duration, whereas others only consider tumour regression sustained for more than three, or even six, months as demonstrating a response. Clearly such variations in the definition of partial response can enormously influence reported response rates in different trials.

Minimal Response

A number of studies have now demonstrated that clinical measurements of anything less than a 50 per cent reduction in tumour size are very unreliable, with enormous observer variation. As a result there is a strong feeling that the category of minimal response, which is based on 50 to 25 per cent tumour shrinkage, should be abandoned as meaningless.

Progression

The problems associated with measurement of tumour shrinkage also apply to increase in tumour size. Criteria for differentiating between disease stabilisation and progression vary widely in different series and hence significantly influence reported failure rates for individual drugs.

Palliation

Palliation, the relief of distressing symptoms, is an important part of cancer treatment but it is difficult to measure as it is usually a subjective evaluation. In the past it has usually been determined either indirectly, the assumption being that if there was tumour shrinkage then symptomatic relief would automatically follow, or by using physical rating scales. The latter have been based on the index of physical performance originally suggested by Karnofsky and Burchenal, in 1948 (see Table 9.1). Although such scales have the virtues of speed and simplicity they may be criticised for concentrating on purely physical status, for ignoring specific symptoms and for relying on an observer's assessment rather than the patient's own opinion.

Recognition of the considerable subjective toxicity of many chemotherapeutic regimes stimulated efforts during the 1970s to develop better

Table 9.1. The Karnofsky index. (Karnofsky D. Burchenal JH (1941). In Clinical Evaluation of Chemotherapeutic Agents in Cancer, ed. Macleod CM. Columbia University Press, New York, p. 191.)

10	Normal
9	Minor signs or symptoms
8	Normal activity with effort
7	Unable to continue normal activity but cares for self
6	Requires occasional assistance with personal needs
5	Disabled
4	Requires considerable assistance and medical care
3	Severely disabled and in hospital
2	Very sick: active supportive treatment necessary
1	Moribund

measures of subjective response and a number of techniques have been developed which are being increasingly used both to determine the relative toxicities of different drugs or treatment regimes and also the subjective benefits of treatment. These techniques include visual rating scales, verbal rating scales and treatment diaries. At present the reliability and relevance of these instruments is still being investigated, but as they are forming an increasingly important part of clinical trial assessments a brief mention of each system is appropriate here.

Visual Rating Scales

These employ the standard psychological method of linear analogue self assessment. The technique is as follows: in order to answer a given question, for example "How tired do you feel today?", a 10cm line is drawn and the ends of the line labelled with the extremes of that parameter, in this case "Not at all" and "Very tired indeed". The patient is then asked to mark on the line where he feels he falls between the two extremes. The distance along the line from one end to the patient's mark may then be measured and a score out of 10 obtained. By compiling proformas made up of a number of relevant questions and asking the patient to complete these at various intervals one may obtain a record of subjective response and toxicity.

Verbal Rating Scales

In this system questions are asked but instead of recording the response by marking a measured line a patient is asked to select from a list of written phrases the one that best describes his situation. Thus in order to answer the question "How tired do you feel today?", some four to seven options would be available such as "Not at all", "Just a little", "Quite tired" and "Very tired indeed".

Diaries

These use a slightly different approach in that patients are given cards marked out in the time scale of their treatment, on which they are asked to record whether certain possible side effects occurred and to note the degree of severity of any symptoms encountered.

Conclusion

If the results of clinical evaluation indicate that the new agent offers a potential benefit, either in terms of improved efficacy or reduced toxicity, then the Product Licence Application or New Drug Approval is submitted. If these are accepted the drug then becomes commercially available. As this chapter has shown, the degree and complexity of testing involved in taking a drug from its first synthesis to the market place is very considerable and may take many years to complete. Table 9.2 shows a typical timescale for this process and Table 9.3 gives an indication of the chances of an individual compound successfully completing the various phases of its development and the research and development costs involved at each stage.

Table 9.2. The development of dacarbazine. (Schepartz SA (1976). Cancer Treatment Reports. 60: 123–124)

1959	First synthesis
1960	Accepted for screening by NCI
1964	Accepted for development
1966	Formulation and production
1966	IND filed
1974	NDA filed
1975	NDA approved

Table 9.3. Development of new drug from discovery to market. (Wells N. (1983) Pharmaceutical innovation: recent trends, future prospects. Office of Health Economics, London.)

	Probability of success (%)	R & D cost (£ million)
Drug synthesis	—	14
Screening	0.01	12
Formulation	3	0.3
Preclinical trials	7	51
Initial clinical use	12	0.2
Controlled clinical tests	25	5
Confirmatory trials	50	4
Regulatory affairs	90	2
Total		89.5

In view of the enormous cost and long delays which these figures exemplify, efforts are now being made by the regulatory authorities, working together with the pharmaceutical industry and cancer research organisations, to modify the present testing system in order to speed the evaluation of potential new anticancer compounds.

Section 2
Biological Response Modifiers

Chapter 10

Biological Response Modifiers

Introduction

In 1906 Paul Ehrlich observed that when a cancer was transplanted from one animal to another of the same species, it failed to grow and was apparently destroyed by the new host. This was interpreted as evidence that immune mechanisms could lead to tumour rejection. The animals studied were not, however, genetically similar and thus what Ehrlich had recorded was the general phenomenon of transplant rejection rather than a specific antitumour effect. Despite this setback the possibility of stimulating the host's own defences to recognise malignant tissue as foreign and bring about its destruction has been vigorously pursued over the years. The numerous clinical techniques that have been employed may be classified into the following five categories:

1. Passive immunotherapy: the transfer of serum components, usually antibodies, from one individual to another.

2. Adoptive immunotherapy: the transfer of immunity by lymphoid cells or their products.

3. Active specific immunotherapy: the injection of tumour cells, or extracts of tumour cells, in an attempt to induce immunity. Cancer cells have been removed from the host, inactivated by chemicals, heat or radiation, and then reinjected, but despite numerous clinical trials no consistent benefit has been shown.

4. Local immunotherapy: there have been many reports of regression of individual tumour nodules following intralesional injection of a wide variety of agents with immunomodulatory activity. It is now generally accepted, however, that these responses merely demonstrate the susceptibility of tumour cells to intense local inflammatory reactions rather than representing a significant effect on tumour–host relationships mediated by the immune system.

5. Systemic nonspecific immunotherapy: this relies on the administration of substances with a nonspecific immunomodulatory effect, in the hope that

their stimulation of some component of the immune system will result in tumour destruction. During the 1960s and 1970s there was great clinical interest in this approach with anecdotal reports and non-randomised studies claiming improvement in a number of human tumours following administration of agents such as BCG, mer-BCG (the methanol extract residue of BCG), *Corynebacterium parvum*, levamisole and thymosin. Subsequent randomised prospective trials failed to confirm these results, leading to a general disillusionment with the concept of immunotherapy among many oncologists in the early 1980s.

One minor therapeutic development resulting from this work was the discovery that local injections of *Corynebacterium parvum* appear to be effective in controlling some malignant pleural and peritoneal effusions (see Chapter 8) but this is almost certainly a reflection of a local inflammatory effect rather than a genuine mobilisation of host defences to destroy tumour cells.

In the last few years developments in immunology and in the disciplines of molecular biology and cellular genetics have rekindled interest in possible biological regulation of tumour growth. As these processes and systems embrace a wider area than traditional immunological approaches the term biological response modification (and hence biological response modifiers, for the active principles) has been adopted for this approach to tumour control. The four key areas of current interest in this context are monoclonal antibodies, lymphokines, oncogenes and growth factors.

Monoclonal Antibodies

A number of tumours in mice, and other animals, possess antigens specific to the individual tumour type. When tumour cells bearing these antigens are injected into a normal mouse its B-lymphocytes will be stimulated to produce specific antibodies to the tumour-specifc antigens. In 1975 Kohler and Milstein reported a technique whereby antibody-producing B-lymphocytes could be fused with myeloma cells, which possessed an infinite capacity for replication (Fig. 10.1). The resulting cells, called hybridomas, contained the genetic material of both their parents and so could reproduce indefinitely. If the original B-lymphocyte had previously been stimulated to produce a specific antibody then the hybridoma resulted in a clone of cells that could make limitless quantities of that antibody. If such monoclonal antibodies could be raised against human tumours then a number of therapeutic possibilities would be offered. These include direct attack on the tumour by the antibody or the use of the antibody as a carrier to target lethal substances, such as cytotoxic drugs, radioactive isotopes or naturally occurring toxins (for example, ricin) directly to the cancer cell without damage to normal tissues.

Although the theory of this approach is very attractive there are many problems in its application. Firstly human tumour specific antigens have still

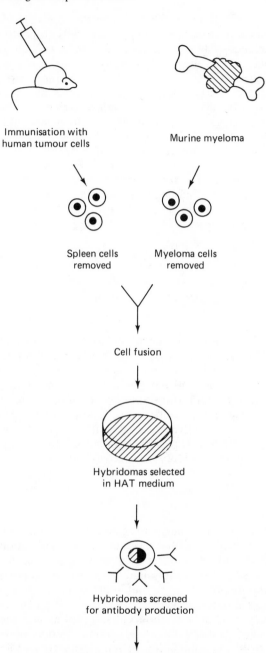

Figure 10.1. Production of monoclonal antibodies. HAT medium contains hypoxanthine, aminopterin and thymidine and only hybridoma cells carry the necessary enzymes to survive in this medium.

to be clearly identified, at best certain antigens have been found which are found in greater concentrations on tumour cells than normal cells – thus the antibodies produced so far are not truly tumour specific. One approach to overcome this problem has been to develop antibodies to tumour products, such as carcino-embryonic antigen (CEA), rather than the cells themselves and to concentrate on using these antibodies as carriers for targeting lethal agents to the tumour as opposed to relying on the antibody itself to be the destructive agent. Furthermore there are still considerable technical difficulties, for example the antibodies raised so far have all been produced in mice and so produce unwanted immune responses when injected into patients: also, the process of producing monoclonal antibodies is still extremely complex and time consuming. For these reasons there have, so far, been relatively few clinical trials with monoclonal antibodies in cancer therapy but occasional responses have been reported. It remains to be seen whether technical refinements can improve results and make this a more practical approach to treatment.

Lymphokines

Lymphokines were originally identified as polypeptide products of certain lymphocytes and were thought to act as molecular signals between different cells within the immune system. It is now clear that these substances may be produced by a variety of different cells and have actions on many tissues within the body; for this reason some authorities are now adopting the term "cytokines" to describe these proteins. A number of different lymphokines have been identified and some have been shown to have anticancer activity. Lymphokines which are currently being explored as potential antitumour agents include interferons, interleukin-2 and tumour necrosis factor.

Interferons

Interferon was first described in 1957 as a substance that could inhibit viral replication but it was not till the early 1980s that production and purification techniques were developed to provide reasonable quantities of material for clinical evaluation. In the intervening years there had been sporadic reports from small series, using very impure preparations, that interferon appeared to have an antitumour, as well as an antiviral, effect.

We now know that there are a number of different interferons and the human forms have been classified as alpha, beta and gamma. Alpha interferons are naturally derived from the stimulation of leukocytes by certain viruses but the development of genetic engineering techniques has allowed the production of clones of bacterial cells producing limitless quantities of alpha-interferon essentially similar to the virally induced form. Beta-interferons are produced by fibroblasts following exposure to viruses and the gamma form was first isolated from lymphocytes following their stimulation by a variety of substances such as phytohaemagglutinin and *Corynebacterium parvum*. To date only alpha-interferons have shown any significant anticancer activity and are the only type of interferon widely available for clinical use.

The precise basis for the antitumour activity of interferons remains uncertain for, as well as having a direct cytotoxic effect, alpha interferon also stimulates a wide range of host defences, in particular a subset of lymphocytes known as natural killer cells, which are thought to play an active part in tumour destruction.

Alpha-interferons have been administered by intravenous, intramuscular and subcutaneous routes with a variety of dose schedules ranging from 3 to 50 mega units daily. Optimum regimes have still to be established and it is not clear whether there is a dose–response relationship. Certainly side effects are greater at higher doses, with anorexia, nausea, tiredness, malaise, myelosuppression, disturbance of liver function tests and neurotoxicity ranging from minor EEG changes and loss of concentration to fits and coma. At lower doses a transient flu-like illness is usually seen after the first few injections, comprising fever, shivering, headache and malaise, but once treatment is established toxicity is generally minimal.

Alpha-interferons are effective agents in an uncommon form of leukaemia – hairy-cell leukaemia – and probably represent the treatment of choice in this condition. They also have activity in renal cell carcinoma, particularly in patients with lung secondaries, some lymphomas and chronic leukaemias, myeloma, malignant carcinoid tumours and malignant melanoma, although their place in the routine management of these conditions has still to be established. Clinical trials to define the role of interferons in cancer treatment are still at an early stage.

Interleukin-2

Interleukin-2 is a protein with a variety of immunomodulatory functions including the activation of a subpopulation of lymphocytes which destroy tumour cells; these lymphocyte-activated killer cells (often abbreviated to LAK-cells) appear to be able to lyse cancer cells which are resistant to the natural killer cells activated by interferons. Several clinical trials have already been carried out with interleukin-2 given either alone or in combination with LAK-cells. Responses have been seen but the treatment is toxic with side-effects including fever, hypotension, hepatic and renal failure, myocardial damage and oedema. Treatment is also extremely expensive and it is far from clear, at present, whether this will prove a useful form of therapy.

Tumour Necrosis Factor

Tumour necrosis factor (TNF or cachectin) is released by mononuclear phagocytes following exposure to endotoxin, and has recently been produced by genetic engineering. Laboratory experiments have demonstrated the ability of TNF to lyse tumour cells, apparently with sparing of normal cells. Clinical evaluation of TNF is at an early stage and has not, so far, been particularly encouraging, with little evidence of response and considerable toxicity. The latter includes fever, hypotension and haemorrhagic necrosis and further research has indicated that TNF may actually be the macrophage hormone released during endotoxic (bacterial) shock and be responsible for mediating many of the clinical symptoms of that condition. For the moment toxicity definitely limits the prospects of this agent becoming part of routine cancer therapy.

Oncogenes

Genes are DNA sequences on the chromosome which control the formation of specific proteins. There is growing evidence that certain genes, or groups of genes, may be involved in the initiation and maintenance of tumour growth. Viruses have long been known to cause a number of cancers in animals and recently specific viral genes leading to tumour formation have been identified. These viral oncogenes have now been found to be virtually identical to certain genes present in normal human cells. The latter have been termed cellular oncogenes (abbreviated to c-onc) or proto-oncogenes. To date some 20 proto-oncogenes have been identified and have been given names such as c-cys, c-fms, c-erb and c-myb.

A number of these proto-oncogenes have been shown to produce proteins which are either growth factors, growth factor receptors or enzymes involved in the initiation of cell division, such as tyrosine kinases (Table 10.1). They are, therefore, thought to have a role in regulating normal cellular proliferation. Evidence is accumulating from a variety of sources that proto-oncogenes also play a part in initiating and maintaining cancer cell growth. Current theories suggest that when these genes are altered by radiation, chemicals or other mutagenic agents, they become oncogenic, either as a result of some structural change or simply due to excessive production

Table 10.1. Some viral oncogenes and the equivalent human proto-oncogenes and their products

Viral oncogene	Tumour from which it was isolated	Equivalent human proto-oncogene	Proto-oncogene product
v-src	Chicken sarcoma	c-src	Tyrosine kinase
v-fes	Cat sarcoma	c-fes	Tyrosine kinase
v-sis	Monkey sarcoma	c-sis	Platelet derived growth factor
v-erbB	Chicken erythroblastosis	c-erbB	Epidermal growth factor receptor
v-fms	Cat sarcoma	c-fms	Colony simulating factor receptor

(amplification) of the gene – the former mechanism resulting in the production of abnormal growth factors, the latter causing an excessive formation of normal growth stimulants.

At present oncogenes have been identified in about one third of human tumours. Whether this indicates that only some tumours are the result of oncogene activation, or that existing techniques are not sufficiently advanced to detect their role in every case remains to be seen. The discovery of proto-oncogenes opens up new directions for cancer treatment with the possibility of producing monoclonal antibodies, or other agents, which could be directed against either the genes themselves or their products. Whether these possibilities can be realised in clinical practice remains to be seen.

Growth Factors

Growth factors are proteins that stimulate cell division by binding to specific receptors on the cell membrane. Most cells are probably capable of producing growth factors and the majority have membrane receptors for several different factors, suggesting that more than one growth factor is necessary to stimulate a specific cell to divide. The multiplicity of growth factors available and the need for several different factors to stimulate any one cell type provide a mechanism for the fine regulation of normal cell growth.

A number of proteins which appear to be involved in the regulation of normal cell growth have now been identified. These include platelet derived growth factor, which plays a part in wound healing as well as cell division, and epidermal growth factor. It is also now clear that many tumour cells produce growth factors and recent studies of the structure of these polypeptides indicate that they are closely related to growth factors found in normal

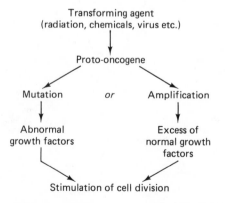

Figure 10.2. Summary of possible relationship between proto-oncogenes, growth factors and cancer formation.

tissues. As we have seen, these growth factors are probably the products of proto-oncogenes.

Once again the discovery and isolation of growth factors provide new alternatives for cancer treatment, with the search for monoclonal antibodies or other agents that will inactivate growth factors or their receptors or inhibit the intracellular enzymes, released by receptor activation, which ultimately cause cell division. As yet the practical therapeutic applications of these discoveries remain largely unexplored but undoubtedly this will be a major area for clinical cancer research over the next decade.

Section 3

The Principles of Endocrine Therapy

Chapter 11

The Development and Rationale of Endocrine Therapy

Introduction

Cellular proliferation in certain organs is influenced by specific hormones. Thus oestrogen will stimulate the growth of the duct system within the female breast and withdrawal of androgens will lead to shrinkage of the prostatic epithelium in men. In 1896 George Beatson, a Scottish surgeon, reported regression of tumour in two premenopausal patients following removal of their ovaries (Beatson G T, Lancet, 2: 104–107, 1896). This observation predated the isolation of oestrogen by some thirty years but was a striking demonstration that malignant tissues as well as normal cells might be sensitive to hormonal influences. It is now clear that a significant proportion of carcinomas of the breast, prostate and endometrium display such hormonal sensitivity and that alteration of the endocrine environment of these cancers may bring about a remission. The initial development of such endocrine therapy was largely empirical and relied on both ablative procedures (where an endocrine organ was surgically excised or destroyed by irradiation, thereby removing the source of a particular hormone) or additive treatment (the administration of natural or synthetic hormones or hormonal antagonists). In the last two decades significant progress has been made in understanding the cellular mechanisms underlying the hormonal sensitivity of cancer. Most of this work has been done on carcinoma of the breast, but the principles which have been established have considerable relevance to a number of other tumours.

The Cellular Basis for Hormonal Sensitivity in Breast Cancer

In the late 1960s it was demonstrated that cells from a number of breast cancers carried receptors for the hormone oestrogen. It soon became clear that the presence of these receptors correlated with a response to endocrine therapy. Subsequently progesterone receptors were also identified and it was shown that if a cell carried both oestrogen receptors (ER+) and progesterone receptors (PgR+) then the chances of a remission with hormonal treatment were further increased. Conversely, receptor negative tumours showed little evidence of hormonal sensitivity (Table 11.1).

Table 11.1.   The relationship between receptor status and response to endocrine therapy. (Table based on pooled data from 10 published series)

Receptor status	Proportion of patients with that status	Incidence of response
ER+PgR+	38%	73%
ER+PgR−	33%	34%
ER−PgR−	26%	10%
ER−PgR+	3%	50%

It has subsequently been shown that a number of breast cancer cells also carry receptors for certain growth factors, including epidermal growth factor and a number of transforming growth factors. It is clear that there is a relationship between oestrogen receptors, growth factor receptors and the secretion of growth factors by tumour cells. The full details of this relationship remain to be clarified, but some aspects are reasonably well defined and suggest a working hypothesis to explain the interaction.

When an oestrogen receptor is stimulated there are two possible consequences, either the formation and release of growth factors, which stimulate the cell to divide, or the production of progesterone receptors, which do not provoke replication and are seen as a move towards greater differentiation of the cell, essentially reducing its malignant potential. Laboratory studies show an inverse correlation between oestrogen receptors (ER) and growth factor receptors (GFR), so that cells with a high ER content have few GFRs and vice versa. It has also been shown that when growth factors are produced they reduce the concentration of ER within the cell as well as stimulating division. Why oestrogen will stimulate some receptors to produce growth factors, which will increase malignancy by stimulating mitosis and reducing ER levels, whilst others are stimulated to produce progesterone receptors, with a consequent decrease in malignancy, is uncertain but it may be related to hormonal concentrations – it has been shown that low levels of oestrogen tend to favour growth factor synthesis whereas higher levels are needed for progesterone receptor formation. The object of hormonal therapy is, therefore, to prevent ER formation of growth factors and encourage ER production of PgR. The mechanisms by which currently available agents might achieve this result are discussed in Chapter 12.

In trying to understand the clinical events seen following endocrine treatment it must be remembered that most tumours will be heterogenous: some clones of cells will be ER+ and PgR+, others will be ER+ and PgR−

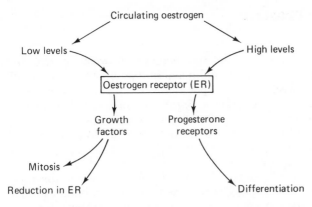

Figure 11.1. Summary of the interaction between free circulating oestrogen and oestrogen receptors.

and others will be ER− and PgR− (as would be expected the combination of ER− and PgR+ is very uncommon). The overall response of the tumour will depend on the relative proportions of these different subsets of cells.

Clinical Correlations of Oestrogen Receptor Status

Assays for the ER content of tumour tissue are now widely available and are used in many centres as a guide to selecting appropriate treatment. As a predictive test the ER assay is useful but not infallible: some ER+ tumours will not respond to endocrine manipulation whilst some ER− cancers will (Table 11.1). Results from numerous clinical trials monitoring receptor status are now available, however, and do permit some general conclusions to be drawn, as follows:

1. Both the proportion of patients who are ER+ and the ER concentrations increase with increasing age. Once an allowance is made for age then menopausal status does not predict for ER status.

2. Incidence and concentration of PgRs is independent of both age and menopausal status.

3. There is no correlation between ER status and the degree of axillary lymph node involvement.

4. The influence of receptor status on overall survival is unclear although there is considerable evidence to suggest that ER+ patients have a longer disease-free interval (the time from primary treatment until evidence of recurrence or metastasis) than those who are ER−.

5. ER status does not predict for response to cytotoxic therapy.

6. Receptor status may change with the natural history of the disease; thus a primary ER+ lesion may recur with ER− metastases, and vice versa.

Carcinoma of the Prostate

The growth of prostatic epithelium and the secretion of prostatic fluid are dependent upon adequate levels of androgen in the blood. Almost all prostatic cancers in man arise from the epithelium. On the assumption that malignant epithelial tissue might retain a degree of androgen dependence Huggins and his colleagues, in the United States, carried out a series of orchidectomies, removing the principal source of androgens, in patients with carcinoma of the prostate. This classic work was reported in 1941, 18 out of 20 men showing an initial improvement with four still alive after five years (Huggins C et al, Archives of Surgery, 43: 209–216, 1949). At about this time the first oestrogens were successfully synthesised and it was demonstrated that they too could control prostatic cancer, offering an alternative form of endocrine therapy in this condition. Both these treatments bring about remissions of 18 to 24 months in some 80 per cent of patients with metastatic disease. Alternative therapies currently being assessed are anti-androgens, such as cyproterone acetate and LHRH agonists (see Chapter 12).

In comparison to carcinoma of the breast the rationale for endocrine therapy in prostatic cancer is very straightforward: the object of treatment is androgen inhibition. Androgen receptors have been identified in prostatic carcinomas but their detection and quantification is far more difficult and less reliable than that of oestrogen receptors in breast cancer. As the great majority of patients will show an objective response to androgen blockade and as no particularly effective cytotoxic therapy is available as an alternative for this predominantly elderly group of patients there has been little motivation to develop routine assays for receptors in these tumours.

Endometrial Carcinoma

The normal endometrium is under two main hormonal influences between the onset of puberty and the menopause. Following menstruation oestrogen secretion leads to proliferation of the endometrium. The addition of proges-terone, secreted by the corpus luteum (which also takes over oestrogen secretion) from about the seventeenth day of the menstrual cycle, leads to maturation of the endometrium with differentiation of supporting cells and secretion of glycogen by the glandular epithelium.

A possible association between hyperplasia of the endometrium and cancer formation was suggested at the beginning of this century. In 1949 it was demonstrated that a progressive series of changes could be seen in the endometrium, giving a continuous spectrum from cystic hyperplasia through to invasive adenocarcinoma. In 1956 it was demonstrated that the earlier changes of this progression could be stimulated in normal women by the administration of large doses of oestrogen. These results, together with data from a number of other sources, form the basis for the current view that carcinoma of the uterine body is, in many cases, the result of the unopposed action of oestrogen on the endometrium. In the late 1950s synthetic progestogens became available and it was argued that their maturing and differentiating action on normal endometrium might be of benefit in adenocarcinoma.

In 1960 the first successful results of progestogen treatment in women with metastatic endometrial carcinoma were reported. Since that time it has been established that some 30 to 40 per cent of patients with advanced disease will gain a remission. This action appears to be the result of a maturing effect of the progestogen on endometrial cancer cells with a reduction in mitotic activity and an increase in glandular differentiation. Treatment is not curative but those who do respond have an average survival a little in excess of 2 years compared to about six months for non-responders. Surgery and radiotherapy result in cure rates of some 80 per cent for primary carcinoma of the uterine body but certain groups of patients who are at risk of recurrence or metastasis can be identified and a number of studies are in progress to assess the role of adjuvant progestogen therapy in early disease.

Normal endometrium contains progesterone receptors, although their concentration varies during the menstrual cycle. Receptors are also seen in some 80 per cent of endometrial hyperplasias and about 60 per cent of adenocarcinomas. The presence of receptors appears to correlate with a response to progestogen therapy but this relationship has not been as extensively explored as that in breast cancer.

Renal Cell Carcinoma

Prolonged administration of oestrogen to male hamsters results in the development of adenocarcinomas of the kidney very similar to those seen in man. This observation, combined with the knowledge of the benefits of progestogen therapy in endometrial cancer, led to a trial of progestin therapy in patients with metastatic renal carcinoma. Although early results were encouraging it is doubtful whether the overall response rate reaches 10 per cent. Until recently there was no other systemic therapy for this condition and so a trial of progestins was always worthwhile, but it is now clear that interferon is useful in this condition, particularly for patients with lung involvement. For those with pulmonary secondaries interferon is the treatment of choice, but in other situations the relative lack of toxicity of progestins means that a trial of therapy is always worthwhile.

Oestrogen or progesterone receptors have been identified in up to 50 per cent of human renal cell carcinomas and it has been claimed that a high receptor content correlates with a response to progestins but receptor assays are not routinely used in the management of this tumour.

Carcinoma of the Thyroid Gland

Adequate primary treatment for a carcinoma of the thyroid gland entails complete destruction of the gland by surgery and radiotherapy. This means that thyroxine secretion is abolished and oral replacement therapy is necessary to prevent the development of myxoedema.

In certain cases oral thyroxine plays a therapeutic as well as a physiological role. In the late 1930s it was noted that prolonged overstimulation of the thyroid gland in rats by thyroid stimulating hormone (TSH), from the anterior pituitary, resulted in the development of thyroid cancers. Since that time there has been much speculation about the role of TSH in the aetiology of human thyroid cancer. There is some evidence that it is a factor in the development of papillary carcinomas. Complete ablation of the thyroid gland results in a fall in blood thyroxine levels which in turn leads to an increase in TSH secretion. If any residual thyroid tissue exists, or if distant metastases are present, then they may well be stimulated by this excessive TSH secretion, especially if the primary tumour was a papillary carcinoma. The administration of oral thyroxine will inhibit TSH release and minimise this risk. Thus thyroid "feeding" has a dual role in prophylaxis, preventing both tumour recurrence and myxoedema. Anaplastic carcinomas show no evidence of TSH dependence and follicular carcinomas very little, but patients with papillary carcinomas who present with advanced disease may often achieve long remissions simply with oral thyroxine therapy.

Glucocorticoids and Cancer Therapy

The cortex of the adrenal gland produces three groups of hormones: the mineral corticoids (regulating sodium balance), the sex hormones (androgens, oestrogens and progesterone) and the glucocorticoids. The glucocorticoids are so called because of their role in regulating carbohydrate metabolism, but they have many other actions in the body including the stimulation of protein metabolism, an anti-inflammatory effect and immunosuppressive properties. The secretion of glucocorticoids is controlled by adrenocorticotrophic hormone (ACTH) which is released by the anterior pituitary gland. The most important naturally occurring glucocorticoids are cortisone and hydrocortisone, the most widely used synthetic preparation is prednisone. Prednisone and related compounds play an important part in the management of cancer, both in the treatment of specific tumours and in the relief of various complications of malignant disease.

Conditions where glucocorticoids play a part in the treatment of the tumour itself are the leukaemias and lymphomas, carcinoma of the breast and brain tumours. The beneficial effects of ACTH in leukaemias were noted as long ago as the 1930s and glucocorticoids used as single agents will produce brief remissions in a number of haematological cancers. Specific glucocorticoid receptors have now been identified in a number of leukaemias and lymphomas. These appear to be commoner in acute leukaemias and high receptor levels do correlate with a response to corticosteroid therapy. Poor concentrations of receptors indicate a lack of response to steroids alone, but the efficacy of combinations of steroids and cytotoxics does not seem to be altered. It is probable that receptor binding is only a partial explanation of steroid acitivity in these tumours and that other, as yet undetermined, factors also play a part. About 10 per cent of patients with advanced breast cancer will benefit from steroid therapy and some breast cancers have been shown to carry glucocorticoid receptors, but the relationship between the presence of receptors and response is uncertain. It has also been suggested that corticosteroids might act by reducing ACTH secretion and thereby lowering circulating oestrogen levels. Alternatively the remissions seen may simply reflect the anti-inflammatory effect of prednisone that results in a reduction of the oedema and inflammation which invariably surrounds tumour deposits. Certainly this is now considered to be the explanation for the beneficial effect seen in many primary and secondary brain tumours following corticosteroid administration.

A number of complications of malignant disease are controlled by the use of corticosteroids. These include hypercalcaemia, some forms of haemolytic anaemia, cerebral oedema and chemotherapy-induced emesis. In addition prednisone frequently has a beneficial subjective effect, with stimulation of appetite, increase in energy and euphoria, which may be valuable in the management of patients with very advanced disease.

Chapter 12

The Clinical Pharmacology of Endocrine Drugs

Anti-oestrogens

Tamoxifen

At least three agents with anti-oestrogenic properties have been used in cancer treatment: tamoxifen, clomiphene citrate and nafoxidene. It is tamoxifen, however, that has come to dominate this particular therapeutic area and the remainder of this discussion will be confined to this agent.

Tamoxifen is a synthetic compound, originally identified during research into novel oral contraceptive preparations, which was subsequently found to have activity in breast cancer. Current understanding of its mode of action in this condition may be summarised as follows: the two principal effects of tamoxifen appear to be an anti-oestrogenic action, resulting from competitive binding with oestrogen receptors (ER) and a weak oestrogen-like effect which results in increased blood levels of sex hormone binding globulin. This latter protein binds to circulating oestrogen and an increase in its concentration reduces the amount of free oestradiol available to bind with ER in tumour cells. Tamoxifen binding with ER prevents the synthesis and release of growth factors but appears to stimulate ER-mediated synthesis of progesterone receptors. The net effect of these actions is inhibition of cell division with arrest at the G_1 stage of the cell cycle. This tamoxifen blockade is reversible and when the concentration of the drug falls the ERs are released and cell growth resumes.

Tamoxifen's action in reducing free circulating oestradiol levels inhibits the negative feedback mechanism for oestrogens to regulate the release of follicle stimulating hormone (FSH) from the pituitary gland. This results in increased FSH levels which will stimulate ovarian production of oestrogens. This process has been cited as a theoretical argument against the use of tamoxifen in premenopausal women. In practice, however, response rates seen in premenopausal breast cancer patients appear similar to those reported in older age groups.

Tamoxifen has emerged as first line therapy for recurrent or metastatic breast cancer. It is being increasingly used in adjuvant therapy of early

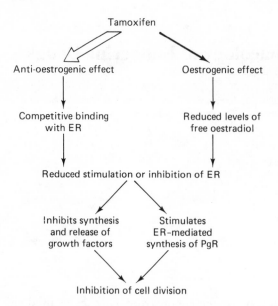

Figure 12.1.   Mechanism of action of tamoxifen.

disease and its possible role in the prevention of breast cancer is being explored. It has been used in other tumours where oestrogen receptors have been isolated, including malignant melanoma and carcinoma of the pancreas, but the results have been disappointing. The usual dose is 20mg daily and randomised studies have failed to show any increase in response rates, response duration or decreased time to response with either higher daily doses or initial loading doses. It has been suggested, however, that patients who relapse after tamoxifen-induced remission may get a further benefit if the

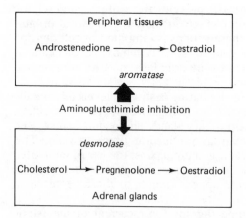

Figure 12.2.   Mechanism of action of aminoglutethimide.

dose is escalated; this remains to be confirmed. In those patients who have responded initially to the drug and then relapse simply stopping tamoxifen administration will bring about a further remission in 15 to 20 per cent of patients – the so-called tamoxifen-withdrawal response.

Side effects of tamoxifen are relatively uncommon and generally mild. They include hot flushes, nausea, dizziness and vaginal bleeding. Fluid retention, thrombocytopenia (mild and transient) and retinopathy are very rare complications of treatment. In a few patients there is a brief worsening of the disease at the start of tamoxifen therapy and in those with bone secondaries acute hypercalcaemia may develop, paradoxically this reaction, termed tamoxifen-flare, usually heralds a good response to the drug.

Inhibitors of Steroid Synthesis

Aminoglutethimide

This drug prevents steroid synthesis by two different mechanisms. It is an inhibitor of the desmolase enzyme system which mediates the initial stages of steroid hormone synthesis in the adrenal glands. It also arrests the action of aromatase, an enzyme found in peripheral tissues, which converts androgen to oestradiol. Initially the adrenal action was thought to be the more important and the phrase "medical adrenalectomy" was often used to describe aminoglutethimide's mode of action. It has subsequently been realised that peripheral conversion of androstendione forms the major source of oestrogen in post-menopausal women and also that aminoglutethimide is a much more powerful aromatase inhibitor than adrenal inhibitor. A very practical consequence of these observations is that the drug may be given in lower doses than those originally recommended with a consequent reduction in toxicity. Aminoglutethimide does not affect ovarian oestrogen production and it is therefore of no value in premenopausal women.

Aminoglutethimide is used in the management of advanced breast cancer; it has also been used in metastatic prostatic carcinoma as second-line therapy following oestrogens or castration and occasional responses have been seen. Aminoglutethimide is derived from the hypnotic agent glutethimide and in consequence is associated with central nervous system side effects including drowsiness, lethargy, dizziness and ataxia. Skin rashes developing during the first few days of drug administration are also common although they usually resolve spontaneously with continued therapy. Severe thrombocytopenia is a rare complication of treatment. Initially the drug was given at a dose of 1G daily and hydrocortisone 20-40mg daily was also given to counteract the aminoglutethimide blockade of glucocorticoid hormone synthesis in the adrenal glands. Subsequently it has been shown that a dose of 125mg twice daily is sufficient to inhibit peripheral oestrogen formation without significant adrenal suppression. At this dose side effects are less severe and less frequent but their incidence is reduced still further if hydrocortisone supplements are retained and so the two drugs are usually given in combination.

Oestrogens

Naturally occurring oestrogens are unsuitable for therapeutic use as they are rapidly metabolised by the liver but a number of synthetic preparations have been employed in the management of advanced cancers of the prostate and breast since the 1950s. Oestrogen administration in men inhibits the release of LH from the anterior pituitary with a consequent fall in testicular androgen production. It may also have a direct effect on prostatic tissue, though the mechanism for this is unclear. The explanation for oestrogen's activity in advanced breast cancer is also uncertain. At low, physiological, doses oestrogen administration stimulates receptors and tumour growth but at higher doses remissions are seen in ER+ patients. A possible explanation is that the higher concentrations of oestrogen resulting from therapeutic administration switch ER activity to progesterone receptor formation and increased differentiation rather than growth factor production thereby inducing a clinical response.

Oestrogen administration is not without its hazards and significant toxic effects include fluid retention, which may lead to oedema, hypertension and cardiac failure. Thromboembolic complications are also common. Nausea and vomiting occurs in about 50 per cent of patients and hypercalcaemia may be precipitated at the start of therapy. In women nipple pigmentation develops and growth of the endometrium is stimulated and as a result vaginal bleeding during treatment is not uncommon. When treatment is stopped withdrawal bleeding, resembling a normal heavy menstrual period, occurs in the majority of patients and is very worrying if no warning of its likelihood has been given. In men there is loss of libido, impotence, shrinkage of genitalia and some degree of proliferation of breast tissue resulting in gynaecomastia.

Synthetic oestrogens in common use include diethyl stilboestrol, which is usually given at a dose of 1 to 5mg daily for prostatic cancer and 5mg tds for breast cancer, ethinyl oestradiol, given orally at 0.1 to 0.5mg tds and phosphorylated methylstilboestrol (Honvan). This latter agent was designed specifically for use in prostatic carcinomas as it is inert until the action of phosphatase enzymes releases free stilboestrol. As prostatic tumours are rich in phosphatases it was thought that use of this agent might lead to selective concentration of oestrogen in the prostate. There is no evidence, however, that it is superior to stilboestrol in this condition although it has been suggested that as it is given intravenously, in doses of 250 to 500mg daily, it may relieve bone pain more quickly than oral preparations.

Androgens

Various androgenic preparations were introduced in the 1950s and played a valuable part in the management of advanced breast cancer until the development of less toxic agents such as the anti-oestrogens. The side effects include fluid retention (less frequently than oestrogens) and hypercalcaemia (more frequently then with oestrogens) but often the most distressing aspect of their administration is virilisation. They do, however, have an anabolic effect often leading to an increase in appetite and a feeling of well being which may be beneficial in some patients. Early preparations were based on testosterone and had the additional hazard of occasional cholestatic jaundice. Later a number of less virilising agents, the anabolic steroids, were developed, including nandrolone (Durabolin) and drostanolone propionate (Masteril) but masculinisation still occurred and limited their usefulness.

Anti-androgens

Cyproterone Acetate (Androcur, Cyprostat)

Cyproterone acetate is a steroidal derivative of hydroxyprogesterone and binds to progesterone receptors. In addition it competes with testosterone for androgenic receptors, thereby blocking the effects of testicular and adrenal androgens. Furthermore the progestogenic actions of the drug reduce LH production by the pituitary, which in turn reduces testicular androgen synthesis.

Cyproterone acetate has been used as an alternative to stilboestrol in the management of prostatic cancer and appears to give similar rates of response. It is less toxic than stilboestrol. Side effects include impotence, tiredness, depression, gynaecomastia and fluid retention but when these do occur they are seldom severe. A typical dose regime is 200 to 300mg daily, by mouth.

Flutamide

This is a non-steroidal agent which prevents testosterone from binding to nuclear receptors in the prostate. In contrast to cyproterone acetate it has no effects on pituitary function or other hormonal systems and has therefore been termed a pure anti-androgen. It has been used in prostatic cancer and appears to have similar activity to stilboestrol. Although it has no effect on libido or potency it does have a number of troublesome side effects including depression, nausea, vomiting and dizziness. Liver damage has also been reported. It is given orally at a dose of 250mg three times daily.

LHRH Analogues

Luteinising hormone-releasing hormone (LHRH) is a decapeptide, produced by the hypothalamus, which binds to receptors in the anterior pituitary gland and stimulates the synthesis and release of luteinising hormone (LH) and follicle stimulating hormone (FSH). A number of synthetic analogues to LHRH have now been prepared and their administration results in an initial increase in LH and FSH levels in the blood but continued therapy appears to reduce the number of LHRH receptors in the pituitary so that within about two weeks gonadotrophin (LH and FSH) levels fall to those seen in castrated patients. As a consequence oestrogen and androgen formation is suppressed with a corresponding fall in their circulating blood levels.

Three LHRH analogues have been assessed in cancer treatment: goserilin acetate (Zoladex: the only agent commercially available in Britain at present), leuprolide (Lupron: available in the USA) and buserilin. Extensive studies in carcinoma of the prostate indicate that these agents produce response rates equivalent to those seen with oestrogen therapy but with less toxicity. Use of the drugs results in a transient rise in androgen levels during the first few weeks of treatment and in those patients where an exacerbation of symptoms might be dangerous (for example, early spinal cord compression due to bone secondaries) the use of an anti-androgen for the first three weeks of treatment is recommended. It is not clear whether this so-called "total androgen blockade" improves the long-term results of treatment. LHRH analogues are also being evaluated in advanced breast cancer, where a number of responses have been seen. Side effects include hot flushes, which occur in about 50 per cent of patients, and loss of libido. Gynaecomastia, nausea and fluid retention are uncommon complications of treatment. Goserilin acetate is given as a depot injection into the subcutaneous tissue of the anterior abdominal wall at a dose of 3.6mg every 28 days. Leuprolide is given by daily subcutaneous injection at a dose of 1mg each day.

The Progestins

Progesterone is secreted by the corpus luteum in the ovary during the latter half of each menstrual cycle. It is also secreted by the placenta during pregnancy. Its principal action is to cause maturation of the endometrium in preparation for receiving the fertilised ovum. Progesterone itself is not used in clinical practice as it cannot be given orally and synthetic preparations are more potent.

The mechanism of action of progestational agents in hormonally sensitive cancers is still incompletely understood but in breast and endometrial carcinomas the anti-oestrogenic action of these drugs is probably their most important effect. At the level of the cancer cell this anti-oestrogenic activity comprises both a reduction in the number of oestrogen receptors and an increase in the enzyme 17β-hydroxysteroid dehydrogenase. The latter converts potent oestradiol to less active oestrone and thus reduces the amount of free oestradiol available within the cell for receptor stimulation. There is also an effect due to stimulation of progesterone receptors leading to differentiation and maturation of the cell with a consequent inhibition of mitosis. In addition the progestins appear to have a direct inhibitory effect on ovarian and adrenal sex hormone production as well as an indirect effect due to reduction in pituitary gonadotrophin levels. As well as this spectrum of endocrinological changes there is also some evidence for a direct cytotoxic effect of progestins on cancer cells.

Although some thirty different synthetic progestins have been prepared only two are widely used in cancer therapy today: medroxyprogesterone acetate (Farlutal, Provera) and megestrol acetate (Megace). The principal side effect of medroxyprogesterone acetate is weight gain. Adrenergic effects, characterised by sweating, muscle cramps and fine tremors may also occur as may corticoid-like effects with fluid retention and moon facies. Medroxyprogesterone acetate also appears to enhance blood clotting mechanisms increasing the risk of complications in patients with known thrombo-embolic disease. Megestrol acetate also causes weight gain and is sometimes associated with nausea, urticaria, carpal tunnel syndrome, thrombophlebitis and alopecia. All progestins may cause gynaecological side effects including vaginal bleeding, amenorrhoea and changes in cervical secretions. Medroxyprogesterone acetate is usually given orally at doses of up to 1 gramme per day, although intramuscular preparations are also available. Megestrol acetate is given at a dose of 160–320mg per day, by mouth.

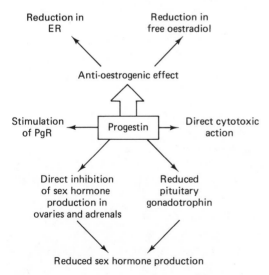

Figure 12.3.   The spectrum of activity of progestins.

The Glucocorticoids

The mechanism of action of the glucocorticoids has been considered in Chapter 11. The side effects of corticosteroid therapy are numerous and frequently severe, they are summarised in Table 12.1. The relative potencies and dosage ranges for some of the preparations in common use are shown in Table 12.2.

Table 12.1. Possible side effects of glucocorticoid therapy

---

1. Suppression and atrophy of adrenal gland

2. Sodium and water retention leading to:
   a. potassium depletion
   b. weight gain
   c. cardiac failure

3. Increased risk of infection

4. Cushingoid appearance:
   a. moon face
   b. buffalo hump

5. Gastrointestinal disturbance:
   a. dyspepsia
   b. peptic ulceration
   c. perforation

6. Osteoporosis

7. Hyperglycaemia

8. Psychosis

9. Skin changes:
   a. thinning of skin
   b. bruising
   c. acne

10. Cataract formation

11. Myopathy

Table 12.2. Relative potencies and typical doses of natural and synthetic glucocorticoids

	Relative potency		Typical daily dose (mg)[a]
	Glucocorticoid activity	Mineralocorticoid activity	
Hydrocortisone	1	1	10–20
Cortisone	0.8	1	10–20
Prednisone	4	0.8	15–60
Prednisolone	4	0.8	15–60
Dexamethasone	25	0	2–16

[a] Hydrocortisone and cortisone are usually only used as replacement therapy in cases of adrenal insufficiency secondary to treatment, for example in patients taking aminoglutethimide: the doses given here are those for this indication. The doses of prednisone, prednisolone and dexamethasone are those which are used in active treatment of tumours.

Section 4

The Clinical Role of Chemotherapy

Chapter 13

The Place of Chemotherapy in Cancer Treatment

Introduction

Most of the major developments in cancer therapy over the last 25 years have been in the field of drug treatment. The advances have frequently been dramatic and impressive, with cure now possible in a number of previously uniformly fatal conditions, such as acute leukaemia, advanced lymphoma, a number of childhood malignancies, metastatic testicular cancer and choriocarcinoma. The fact that these tumours very often affect young people has made these successes all the more important and emotive. Unfortunately, however, cancers curable with chemotherapy form only a small proportion, less than 10 per cent, of all malignant tumours and it is the older, perhaps less glamorous, modalities of surgery and radiotherapy which still account for the great majority of cancer cures today. This is especially true in the solid tumours, the carcinomas and sarcomas, which account for over 90 per cent of cancers, where, with the possible exception of early breast cancer and a few uncommon conditions, chemotherapy has yet to make any significant impact on cure rates or survival times.

It is also important to remember that many of the recent improvements in results have come from combining drug treatment with established therapies. This combined approach to treatment, which recognises that the different modalities available are complementary rather than competitive and mutually exclusive, has been the crucial factor in the improved management of many tumours. To understand the basis for such a collaborative approach it is necessary to consider the relative strengths and weaknesses of the various therapeutic options available.

Advantages and Limitations of Available Treatment Modalities

Surgery is a local treatment and is successful when the cancer is limited to an anatomically accessible site. Its greatest value lies in the treatment of early cancer before spread of the tumour has occurred. Surgical failure may be due to one of two factors. First, inadequate excision resulting in local recurrence of the tumour at the site of resection. This may be the result of difficulty in clearing the disease completely from the anatomical site, transection of clinically undetectable microscopic projections of tumour into the surrounding tissue or implantation of tumour cells into the wound. Second, the local excision may have been complete but treatment fails because the tumour had already metastasised and the patient will relapse as a result of the subsequent growth of occult micrometastases which were clinically undetectable at the time of operation.

Radiotherapy is also a local form of treatment and the reasons for its failures are similar to those of surgery: local recurrence or the growth of metastases which were clinically undetectable at the time of primary treatment. There is, however, one important difference. It is usually possible for the radiotherapy field to cover a wider volume of tissue around the tumour than can be removed surgically. Thus the likelihood of local recurrence occurring as the result of failure to treat the margins of the tumour is much less than with surgery. Local recurrence occurs because of the failure of radiation adequately to sterilise the tumour core. This central area of the growth will contain many viable malignant cells which will be rendered radioresistant as the result of local hypoxia. When treatment is completed these cells will be able to repopulate the tumour.

Chemotherapy is a systemic treatment, drugs enter the bloodstream and reach most parts of the body. Such treatment is of the greatest value in widespread disease, either where the condition is disseminated from the outset, such as the acute leukaemias, or where multiple metastases are present. Successful drug treatment requires that the tumour contains the highest possible proportion of actively dividing cells and that these cells are readily accessible via the bloodstream. These conditions are most likely to be met when tumour deposits are small. The reason for treatment failure is the presence of large masses of tumour made up of a high proportion of resting cells and containing extensive avascular areas harbouring viable cancer cells. Almost invariably drug toxicity or tumour resistance will develop before such large masses may be destroyed.

These factors mean that although many very early lesions may be cured by surgery or radiotherapy alone, when there is a risk of local extension of the disease the chances of cure will be increased if surgery and radiotherapy are combined and if there is a likelihood of distant micrometastases being present then adjuvant chemotherapy should further improve results. The application of these simple principles has been a major factor in the improved results of cancer treatment over the last two decades.

The Objectives of Cancer Treatment

The ultimate goal of cancer treatment is to achieve a cure. Despite advances in therapy in recent years this is still only possible for 35 to 40 per cent of patients. For the remainder the aim must be to gain a worthwhile increase in survival, ensuring not only an enhanced life-expectancy but also a good quality of life during that time, or, when prolongation of life is unattainable, palliation, with prompt relief of distressing symptoms, is the goal.

Although these aims are easily stated Chapter 8 has already shown the difficulties encountered in trying to measure the extent to which they are met by individual treatment policies. These difficulties are compounded in the rapidly developing field of cancer chemotherapy since new drugs and new techniques for improving the results from existing agents are continually being introduced. But cancer chemotherapy is often extremely toxic, occasionally lethal, and frequently highly expensive. Furthermore it is clear that the very dramatic results first seen in a number of highly chemo-sensitive, but uncommon, cancers in the 1960s and 1970s have not been reproduced in most other tumours. The indiscriminate use of chemotherapy will therefore cause much needless toxicity and distress whilst consuming, and wasting, enormous resources and far from enhancing survival may actually reduce it.

Some guidelines must therefore be recognised in order to determine when chemotherapy is indicated in the management of individual cancer patients. Table 13.1 is an attempt to summarise the situation. It is based on data available from clinical trials which have matured during the 1980s. Inevitably some oncologists will see individual recommendations as too conservative whilst others will view them as unduly aggressive. The subsequent chapters are an attempt to explain the background to the table by explaining the place of chemotherapy in specific tumours in a little more detail. Before moving to these discussions some general comments are necessary.

Where chemotherapy is the sole, or major, modality for cure there is obviously no doubt that treatment is mandatory. There are, however, few, if any, cancers where drug treatment offers a 100 per cent cure rate with no side effects. Therefore, even in highly chemosensitive tumours, there is still a need for continuing development in order to improve cure rates and reduce toxicity. Such developments require assessment and so there is still a strong argument for treating most of these patients in the context of planned clinical trials in order to ensure the continued improvement of results.

Such trials are especially important in the many grey areas of chemotherapy where, although responses have been seen, there is still uncertainty as to whether treatment genuinely enhances survival. In addition it is essential that increasing attention is given to the quality and duration of survival and the cost to the patient, in terms of subjective toxicity and general inconvenience, that is entailed in treatment. Also, in these times of limited resources for health care, the economics of therapy must be considered and some responsibility taken for ensuring that therapy is cost-effective.

Such assessments are integrally related to assessment of the quality of survival and such subjective measurements remain controversial and unreliable. One fact that is clear, however, and which relates particularly to the use of chemotherapy in advanced disease, is that the physical performance status of the patient heavily influences the outcome of treatment. Table 13.2 summarises data from studies in advanced gastrointestinal cancer, but similar figures are available for most other tumours, all clearly showing that the

Table 13.1. Summary of the place of chemotherapy in the treatment of cancer

Tumour and its incidence (as a percentage of all cancers)	Chemotherapy is the sole or dominant modality for cure in certain stages of the disease	Chemotherapy may increase survival if given as an adjuvant in early disease	Chemotherapy may increase survival time in advanced disease	Chemotherapy may lead to tumour shrinkage in occasional patients	Chemotherapy has little or no effect
Childhood cancer, 1.5	a				
Acute leukaemia, 0.75	a				
Chronic leukaemia, 1	b				
Hodgkin's disease, 0.75	a		a		
Non-Hodgkin's lymphoma, 2	a		a		
Myeloma, 0.5			a		
Non-small-cell lung cancer, 13				a	
Small-cell lung cancer, 4			a		
Breast cancer, 12		b,c	a,c		
Oesophageal cancer, 2					a
Carcinoma of stomach, 9				a	
Carcinoma of pancreas, 3					a
Colorectal cancer, 13				a	
Anal carcinoma	b				
Renal cell carcinoma, 1				a,d	
Carcinoma of bladder, 3		b		a	
Prostatic carcinoma, 4	a		a,c		
Testicular cancer, 0.5	a				
Carcinoma of uterine cervix, 3		b	b		
Endometrial carcinoma, 2.5		b,c	a,c		
Ovarian cancer, 2.5		b	a		
Choriocarcinoma, <0.1	a		a		
Head and neck cancer, 3				a	
Skin cancer, 10					a
Melanoma, 0.3					a
Brain tumours, 2				a	
Soft tissue sarcoma, 0.5		b	b		
Osteosarcoma		a	a		
Thyroid cancer, 0.5				a,c	a

a Activity established in this category.
b Preliminary results suggest activity in this category but confirmation awaited.
c Endocrine therapy plays a major part.
d Biological response modifiers play a major part.

Table 13.2. The relationship between response to cytotoxic chemotherapy and performance status in patients with advanced gastrointestinal cancer. (Moertel CG (1976). British Journal of Cancer, 34: 325–334)

Performance status	Response rate (%)
Gastric carcinoma	
Fully active, working whole or part time	39
Ambulatory but spends most of the day in bed or in a chair	4
Colorectal carcinoma	
Fully active, working whole or part time	31
Ambulatory but spends most of the day in bed or in a chair	7

better the general condition of the patient the greater the chance of a response.

In selected patients with specific cancers chemotherapy is potentially life-saving but there is no doubt that over the last ten to fifteen years the successes seen in some, very limited, areas have often resulted in indiscriminate treatment of other patients with damaging results not only to individuals but to the reputation of chemotherapy in general. A major part of the expertise of the oncologist is knowing the indications for drug treatment and, perhaps even more importantly, knowing when such treatment is inappropriate.

Chapter 14

Childhood Cancer

Introduction

Childhood cancer is relatively uncommon, affecting about 1 in 650 of those under 15 years of age and accounting for less than 2 per cent of all cancers. It is, however, a very important area of oncology as enormous advances have been made in the treatment of these tumours over the last thirty years and many previously uniformly fatal tumours are now curable in a high proportion of children. Table 14.1 summarises the relative incidence and changing survival rates of the various childhood cancers. The leukaemias, lymphomas and osteosarcoma will be discussed in subsequent chapters.

Table 14.1. Childhood cancers; relative incidence and survival (per cent)

Tumour	Incidence	5-year survival	
		1954–1963	1974–1983
Acute lymphoblastic leukaemia	26	2	47[a]
Other leukaemias	7	2	20[a]
Hodgkin's disease	4	44	90[a]
Non-Hodgkin's lymphoma	5	18	46[a]
Medulloblastoma	5	25	40
Other CNS cancers	18	10–70[b]	20–80[b]
Wilms' tumour	5	30	85[a]
Rhabdomyosarcoma	4	25	55
Ewings' sarcoma	5	10	40
Osteosarcoma	2	15	40[a]
Neuroblastoma	6	14	28[a]
Retinoblastoma	3	80	80
Other cancers	10	–	–
All cases	100	30	50

[a] Results in the 5-year period 1979–83 were better than in 1974–78 suggesting that survival is still increasing in these tumours.
[b] Various tumours, with a wide range of prognoses but no significant improvement in survival has been achieved in any tumour type.

Chemotherapy has been a major factor in the improved cure rates for many of these tumours but improvements in radiotherapy, surgery and supportive care have also played a significant part in increasing survival. Perhaps even more importantly the relative rarity of childhood cancers, together with the complex therapy they require, has meant that these patients have increasingly been managed in specialist regional centres, which have developed multidisciplinary teams specifically devoted to the highly specialised and sophisticated treatment and care that these children require. This concentration of patients and expertise has also meant that a very high proportion of children with cancer are entered into clinical trials and this has undoubtedly greatly increased the speed with which therapeutic innovations have been evaluated and, where appropriate, incorporated into routine treatment.

Wilms' Tumour

Wilms' tumour is an embryonal cancer of the kidney occurring in early childhood, the majority of patients being under 5 years of age. The management of Wilms' tumour has progressed by a series of well documented steps and provides a model for the integration of new therapeutic developments into an overall plan of treatment, with a consequent increase in survival. For this reason Wilms' tumour, although exceedingly uncommon, has a considerable significance for oncologists.

In the early part of this century surgery was the only treatment available and cured about 15 per cent of patients. Improvements in diagnosis and surgical technique raised this figure to 30 per cent by the 1930s. Wilms' tumour proved moderately radiosensitive and the combination of radiotherapy and surgery improved survival to just over 40 per cent by the late 1940s. Usually radiotherapy was given post-operatively to the renal bed but in some instances it was used pre-operatively to reduce tumour size in order to facilitate resection.

In 1957 a number of children with metastatic Wilms' tumour were treated with actinomycin-D. The results were encouraging and the drug was soon being extensively used in children with advanced disease but, although many responses were seen with chemotherapy, there was no evidence of an overall increase in long-term survival.

At presentation, the majority of children have tumour apparently confined to the kidney or renal bed, suitable for treatment with surgery and post-operative radiotherapy. Follow-up of these patients has shown that at least 50 per cent of them have occult metastases, usually in the lungs, present at the time of their initial diagnosis. The realisation that the tumour was sensitive to actinomycin-D and that potentially lethal microscopic secondaries were present in 50 per cent or more of patients at the time of initial treatment led to the introduction of actinomycin-D, given for 5 days in the immediate post-operative period, as adjuvant therapy in patients with apparently localised disease. As a result cure rates rose to over 60 per cent and Wilms' tumour provided the first evidence of the benefits of adjuvant cytotoxic therapy in early malignant disease. Combining vincristine with actinomycin-D and continuing therapy, on an intermittent schedule for 9 to 10 months after resection, has further improved survival to the level shown in Table 14.1.

More recent developments are the addition of doxorubicin to the drug regime and introduction of neo-adjuvant chemotherapy. Doxorubicin has been shown to be active against Wilms' tumour, but it does increase the toxicity of drug treatment. Current protocols are comparing actinomycin-D and vincristine with or without doxorubicin in the more advanced stages of the disease, in order to establish whether the three drug regime does actually increase survival. Rescheduling chemotherapy to start treatment prior to resection has resulted in significant reductions in tumour size, with a consequent improvement in ease of resection. After preoperative cytotoxic treatment some 40 per cent of children have stage I tumours (disease limited to the kidney and completely resectable) as compared to only 20 per cent prior to the introduction of neo-adjuvant therapy. A further benefit of this approach is that post-operative radiotherapy is no longer necessary for many patients.

Current clinical trials in early Wilms' tumour are concentrating on defining the scheduling of actinomycin-D and vincristine in order to identify the best regimes for neo-adjuvant treatment and the optimum duration for post-operative chemotherapy.

Neuroblastoma

Neuroblastoma is a tumour of the sympathetic ganglia and 70 per cent of tumours arise in the retroperitoneal area, in or around the adrenal gland. It is predominantly a disease of early childhood, 50 per cent of the patients being under two years of age. Those who present in infancy, aged one year or less, form about one third of all cases and have a significantly better prognosis than older children, regardless of the disease stage. The natural history of the tumour is paradoxical in that although generally highly aggressive, with about 75 per cent of patients having metastatic disease at presentation, spontaneous cures with maturation of tumour to a benign state are well documented. For most patients with secondary spread, however, the outlook remains poor despite intensive therapy.

When the tumour is localised surgical excision is the treatment of choice and if the resection appears complete then no further therapy is necessary. For larger tumours regional radiotherapy has been used, but it is now clear that cytotoxic therapy can reduce a number of these tumours to a resectable size and this offers an alternative approach to their management. Adjuvant chemotherapy following irradiation or resection of larger tumours does not appear to enhance survival.

Chemotherapy has been extensively used in metastatic disease: cyclophosphamide, vincristine, dacarbazine, doxorubicin, etoposide and cisplatinum have all been shown to have activity as single agents. Current protocols are evaluating four-drug combinations selected from these drugs. Although responses are seen in up to 80 per cent of patients the only evidence of long-term remission, with improved survival, comes from those children under one year of age. In order to try and improve results in older children high-dose melphalan therapy with autologous marrow transplantation has been used but the benefits of this are still uncertain.

Central Nervous System (CNS) Tumours

Tumours of the brain are the second commonest form of cancer in childhood after the leukaemias. The majority of these are either astrocytomas (40 per cent) or medulloblastomas (20 per cent). This latter tumour occurs almost exclusively in childhood and adolescence and is unusual among primary brain tumours in that it may metastasise throughout the CNS. Primary treatment for CNS tumours in children consists of surgery, where possible, followed by irradiation. In the case of medulloblastoma the whole CNS axis, brain and spinal cord, must be treated because of the danger of secondary spread.

Chemotherapy has been largely reserved for recurrent disease and the results are generally a little more encouraging than with adult cancers of the CNS. The combination of CCNU and vincristine has been the most widely used and response rates of up to 70 per cent have been reported in recurrent low grade (good prognosis) astrocytomas. This evidence of activity has prompted the use of this combination as adjuvant therapy following radiation for high-grade (poor prognosis) astrocytomas and medulloblastomas. Initial studies suggest that survival may be improved as a result. In the last few decades, however, the only clear evidence of enhanced survival in paediatric CNS tumours comes from children with medulloblastoma, but this benefit is almost entirely attributable to improvements in radiotherapy rather than chemotherapy.

Rhabdomyosarcoma

Rhabdomyosarcomas are malignant tumours located in striated muscle but arising from primitive embryonic mesenchymal tissue which has never matured, rather than being true tumours of skeletal muscle. They are seen in childhood and adolescence, with two peaks of incidence at about 5 and 18 years, respectively. The tumours occur most commonly in the head and neck, particularly the orbit, and in the urogenital system.

Over the last twenty years, chemotherapy has been the major factor in the improved cure rates for this very aggressive tumour. During the 1960s and 70s cyclophosphamide, ifosfamide, actinomycin-D, doxorubicin, vincristine and cisplatinum were all shown to have activity in metastatic or inoperable rhabdomyosarcoma. Giving combinations of two or three of these drugs and commencing therapy prior to any attempt at local treatment with surgery or irradiation, has resulted in a major improvement in survival. All patients are now routinely given cytotoxic therapy as first line treatment with combinations of ifosfamide, vincristine and actinomycin-D or vincristine, cyclophosphamide and doxorubicin. If, after three courses of these drugs, there is a greater than 50 per cent regression of tumour treatment is continued for a further three courses. If there is still disease present at this stage, or if a 50 per cent response was not achieved after the initial three courses, then an alternative combination is introduced. Local treatment is only used for control of residual disease when chemotherapy cannot achieve a complete response, or where there was originally bulky disease and microscopic deposits might still be present. Defining the precise indications for surgery and radiotherapy after a complete response to chemotherapy, identifying the optimum duration of drug treatment and modifying treatment schedules to try and improve results in specific subgroups of patients are the main objectives of current clinical trials in these tumours.

Ewing's Sarcoma

Ewing's sarcoma is a bone tumour affecting older children and adolescents, the peak incidence being in those between 10 and 15 years. Its cell of origin has been disputed ever since Ewing first described the tumour in 1921. The primary lesion may be readily controlled by either radiotherapy or surgery but if no further treatment is offered the 5-year survival is dismal due to the rapid appearance of metastases, usually in the lungs and bone marrow. It is now recognised that these must be present at the time of diagnosis, although they may not be clinically apparent, and that Ewing's sarcoma should be managed as a systemic disease from the outset, even if the tumour appears localised. As a result, adjuvant cytotoxic therapy has become a routine part of treatment following initial radiotherapy (or, less commonly, surgery) for the primary lesion. This has been the major factor in the improved survival figures shown in Table 14.1.

Cyclophosphamide, vincristine, actinomycin-D, doxorubicin and ifosfamide have all shown activity against Ewing's sarcoma when used as single agents. The first four of these drugs have been routinely used in combination as adjuvant therapy for up to 18 months following initial radiotherapy. As a result, the overall survival has risen from 10 to over 40 per cent. Unfortunately, those patients with tumours arising on the central skeleton, those who have large primaries and those who present with metastases, still have a poor prognosis. Current attempts to improve the treatment of these children include the substitution of ifosfamide for cyclophosphamide, giving high-dose melphalan with autologous bone marrow transplantation and the use of total body irradiation, with autologous marrow transplantation, following standard four-drug cytotoxic therapy. The success of these various measures remains to be determined.

Retinoblastoma

This rare tumour arises from retinal tissue and is virtually confined to children under 5 years of age. At the time of presentation spread of tumour outside the orbit is uncommon and treatment consists of a combination of surgery and radiotherapy. For patients with metastatic disease cyclophosphamide, ifosfamide and doxorubicin have been shown to have activity as single agents and the combination of vincristine, cyclophosphamide, cisplatinum and etoposide has been claimed to give a 60 per cent response rate. There is no evidence of cure as a result of cytotoxic therapy in advanced disease and the role of chemotherapy as an adjuvant to local treatment in earlier stages of the disease has still to be evaluated.

Chapter 15

Haematological Cancers

Introduction

The haematological cancers account for only about 5 per cent of malignancies but cytotoxic therapy plays a major part in their management and has brought about a dramatic improvement in the prognosis for many of these tumours, offering the possibility of cure in a significant number of patients. The haematological cancers are a very diverse group of diseases, the principal members of which are the leukaemias and lymphomas. The leukaemias are characterised by the production of excessive numbers of white blood cells and many different forms of the disease exist. These are classified into four major groups: acute lymphoblastic leukaemia, acute myeloid leukaemia, chronic myeloid leukaemia and chronic lymphoid leukaemia. The lymphomas are primary cancers of the lymphoreticular system: they usually arise in lymph nodes but may originate in any organ containing lymphoid tissue. The disease may remain localised for a variable period of time but, if untreated, all lymphomas will become disseminated and ultimately fatal. The lymphomas are classified under two headings: Hodgkin's disease and the non-Hodgkin's lymphomas. There are a number of other haematological cancers apart from the leukaemias and lymphomas, the two commonest of which are multiple myeloma and polycythaemia vera and these will also be considered in this chapter.

Acute Lymphoblastic Leukaemia

Acute lymphoblastic leukaemia (ALL) is predominantly a disease of childhood and is far the commonest form of cancer in children, with a peak incidence between 2 and 7 years of age. In 1965 less than 1 per cent of patients with ALL achieved long-term survival whereas today the cure rate exceeds 50 per cent. This improvement in the results of treatment has come about because of sequential modifications to therapeutic regimes which have been systematically assessed in prospective randomised clinical trials.

By the early 1960s it was recognised that initial treatment with vincristine and prednisolone could induce remission (disappearance of clinical signs of disease with a reduction of leukaemic cells in the bone marrow to less than 5 per cent) in 80 to 90 per cent of children. Relapse was, however, inevitable and to try and prevent this, additional therapy was given following remission induction. Three types of post-remission chemotherapy, of varying intensity, are now recognised in the management of ALL. These are consolidation (giving further courses of the same, or similar, drugs used for remission-induction, at equivalent doses and hence equivalent toxicity), maintenance (giving prolonged treatment which is less myelosuppressive and less intensive than that employed during induction) and intensification (using the same drugs as those given during induction but at higher doses or using an alternative high-dose aggressive regime).

Initially a relatively short period of consolidation therapy, with drugs like cytosine arabinoside, methotrexate, cyclophosphamide or 6-mercapto-purine, was followed by a much longer period of maintenance therapy, extending for several years, usually giving methotrexate and 6-mercaptopu-rine. It subsequently became clear that the addition of an anthracycline, usually daunorubicin, and asparaginase further enhanced response rates. This offered two alternative strategies: either to use an aggressive approach to induction using four drugs (vincristine, prednisolone, daunorubicin and asparaginase) and to discard consolidation or to use three drugs initially (vincristine, prednisolone and asparaginase) to be followed by consolidation or intensification with combinations such as cyclophosphamide and daunoru-bicin. It is still not clear which is the best approach but what has emerged is that some children need far less aggressive, and hence less toxic, treatment than others to achieve long-term remission. This has resulted in great efforts to try and identify good and bad prognostic factors in order to adjust more specifically the intensity of treatment to meet the needs of individual patients (see below). The need for maintenance therapy in ALL has not been questioned, but the optimum duration of such treatment has still to be determined, although it does appear unlikely that prolonging chemotherapy beyond 2 to 3 years improves cure rates.

In early trials a major cause of failure was relapse within the central nervous system, and as a result CNS prophylaxis has become an essential part of all treatment regimes in order to eradicate leukaemic cells from the craniospinal meninges. Radiotherapy to the whole brain and spinal canal, to a dose of 24 Gray, or cranial irradiation with intrathecal methotrexate have both proved effective prophylactic treatments. Craniospinal irradiation is, however, myelosuppressive and increases the risk of second cancers and marrow relapse, whilst being associated with growth disturbance and intellec-tual impairment, particularly in very young children. There has, therefore, been an increasing move towards lower dose irradiation (18 Gray) of the brain alone combined with intrathecal methotrexate. More recently it has been suggested that intensive intrathecal chemotherapy, with a combination of methotrexate, cytosine arabinoside and hydrocortisone, may allow radio-therapy to be discarded completely.

Initially the search for prognostic factors to identify subgroups of patients which might require more, or less, intensive therapy relied on clinical features such as the white cell count (very high levels at the time of diagnosis carried a poor outlook), age (children under 1 year and adults over 25 years faring worse than those between 1 year and 25 years, with children between 2 years and 10 years doing best) and the presence of CNS involvement at presentation (indicating a poor prognosis). Improvements in treatment have reduced the validity of these indicators, but during the 1970s it became clear that specific subgroups of ALL could be identified by immunological means and related to their cell of origin. Thus four subgroups were identified: common, null-cell, B-cell ALL (these three being derived from B-lymphocytes at various stages of their development) and T-cell ALL (derived from the T-lymphocyte series). The relative frequencies of these forms of ALL are shown in Table 15.1. Overall common or C-ALL responds best to treatment whereas B-cell ALL carries the poorest prognosis. It is also now apparent that these groups may be further subdivided on the basis of certain chromosomal (cytogenetic) abnormalities and that different drugs may have different levels of activity against the various leukaemic subtypes. Thus a great deal of effort is currently being devoted not only to relating immunological and cytogenetic markers to the overall intensity of therapy required but also to determining whether specific drugs and schedules are needed for the optimum treatment of individual subgroups.

Table 15.1. Incidence of immunological subtypes of acute lymphoblastoid leukaemia

Subtype	Incidence (per cent)	
	Children	Adults
Common	76	50
Null-cell	11	38
B-cell	1	2
T-cell	12	10

Acute Myeloid Leukaemia

In contrast to ALL, acute myeloid leukaemia (AML) is predominantly a disease of adults, with a median age of onset in the mid-50s. Great progress has been made in the treatment of AML over the last 30 years and particularly in the last decade. In the mid-1950s the disease was uniformly fatal, with an average survival time of less than 2 months. By the mid-1980s 65 to 70 per cent of patients were achieving complete remission, with apparent cure of at least 25 per cent of those gaining a remission, and the results of treatment are continually improving.

As with ALL, the first stage in treatment is remission induction. The DAT regime (daunorubicin, cytosine arabinoside and 6-thioguanine) has been the most widely used combination and results in complete remissions in 75 per cent of patients under 60 years of age and about 50 per cent of those over 60, giving an overall remission rate of about 65 per cent. The precise dose and scheduling of the three drugs used is being constantly refined and it has recently been suggested that in some protocols a two drug regime (omitting 6-thioguanine) or even high-dose cytosine arabinoside alone, are as effective as the three-drug combination but these observations remain to be confirmed.

A number of clinical studies have compared consolidation regimes, using further courses of DAT, with maintenance therapy, the latter based on four- to six-drug combinations selected from vincristine, prednisolone, cyclophosphamide, doxorubicin and the nitrosoureas in addition to daunorubicin, cytosine arabinoside and 6-thioguanine. As yet, the results are inconclusive but there is a suggestion that there is no advantage to prolonging treatment beyond 8 months after complete remission has been achieved and that the shorter consolidation technique may be the more efficacious. This indication that the shorter, more intensive, regime might be the more beneficial has encouraged the evaluation of intensification protocols. A variety of these regimes are now undergoing evaluation. They are based on a number of different combinations, but the use of high-dose cytosine arabinoside is common to them all. Preliminary results are encouraging, but it is too early to judge whether intensification will displace consolidation or maintenance therapies. A further unknown in the chemotherapeutic management of AML is the ultimate value of a number of the newer cytotoxic agents which have been shown to have activity in the disease. These include mitozantrone, etoposide and amsacrine and studies are currently underway to determine whether they have a place in the routine management of AML.

Bone marrow transplantation offers a different approach to post-remission therapy. The aim here is to ablate the bone marrow with a combination of chemotherapy and radiotherapy (most commonly giving high-dose cyclophosphamide followed by total body irradiation) and then to "rescue" the patient with an infusion of new marrow cells. There are three potential sources for such cells: marrow from an identical twin (a syngeneic transplant), marrow from an immunologically closely compatible donor, usually a sibling (an allogeneic transplant) and marrow harvested from the patient prior to ablation (an autologous transplant). Clearly the chances of a patient with AML having an identical twin are remote and a major problem with autologous transplants is the risk of reintroducing leukaemic cells (although a number of techniques are being evaluated for "cleaning" the patient's marrow, once it has been harvested, in order to remove residual cancer cells). At present, therefore, the main experience of transplantation in AML is based on allogeneic marrow transplants.

The risk of graft-versus-host disease, the toxicity of marrow ablation and the high risk of life-threatening infection during the rescue phase currently restrict consideration of bone marrow transplantation to patients under 45 years old (well below the median age of onset of the disease). Furthermore, in order to minimise the risk of rejection, usually only siblings are considered as donors. Given these limitations, currently only 10 per cent of AML patients are suitable for bone marrow transplantation following remission induction. Recent results show that of those who undergo transplantation 50 per cent or more become long-term survivors and appear to be cured. It is still not clear, however, when allowance has been made for the younger age, and hence better prognosis, of the transplant population, whether these results are really superior to those seen with chemotherapy.

The long-term remissions seen following bone marrow transplantation in AML have led to this technique being explored in other leukaemias and lymphomas. With the possible exception of chronic myeloid leukaemia the results have been generally disappointing.

Chronic Myeloid Leukaemia

Chronic myeloid leukaemia is a generic term which includes a number of different chronic proliferative diseases of the granulopoietic cells of the bone marrow. This discussion will be restricted to chronic granulocytic leukaemia (CGL), which accounts for the great majority of chronic myeloid leukaemias, the other forms being either rare or very rare.

CGL has a peak age incidence between 40 and 60 years but may occur at any time and often affects young adults. 95 per cent of patients with CGL will have an abnormal chromosome, the Philadelphia (Ph) chromosome, present in virtually all their myeloid cells at the time of diagnosis. The natural history of the disease may be divided into three phases. There is an initial chronic phase, which may last some years with little or no evidence of disease progression; a transitional phase of accelerated myeloproliferation, often termed metamorphosis, which is frequently accompanied by anaemia and/or thrombocytopenia and lasts for up to 12 to 18 months, often proving fatal; those who survive metamorphosis go on to develop an invariably fatal acute leukaemia-like terminal phase. Survival times in CGL vary greatly from less than a year to well over 10 years. There is good evidence that active treatment enhances life expectancy; it has been estimated that the average survival time from diagnosis with untreated CGL is 20 months, whereas with current therapy this is increased to 40 to 50 months.

For many years radiotherapy was the treatment of choice for CGL. In America low-dose whole-body irradiation was favoured but in Britain splenic irradiation was the usual practice. Such irradiation not only reduced the spleen size but usually induced a remission in the systemic disease, with a fall in the peripheral white cell count and correction of anaemia. It was subsequently discovered that similar results could be obtained with the alkylating agent busulphan and, in 1968, the Medical Research Council organised a clinical trial to compare busulphan and splenic irradiation in CGL. The mean survival time of irradiated patients was 28 months and that of the group given busulphan 39.5 months. Since these results were published, chemotherapy has tended to displace radiotherapy as the treatment of choice for CGL. Many other drugs have subsequently been shown to have activity in CGL, including melphalan, cyclophosphamide, 6-mercaptopurine, 6-thioguanine and hydroxyurea, but none has proved superior to busulphan which is usually given orally in a dose sufficient to keep the white blood cell count between 10,000 and 20,000 per mm.[3]

Despite the efficacy of busulphan in prolonging survival, cures were never achieved and more aggressive cytotoxic regimes were of little value during the terminal phases of the disease. Recently it has been shown that interferons have activity in CGL and, in contrast to conventional cytotoxics, they not only reduce the number of myeloid cells but actually reduce the proportion of Ph chromosome positive marrow cells, suggesting a more profound effect on the biology of the tumour than simple cell kill. Another new development is the use of bone marrow transplantation in selected patients, using various combinations of chemotherapy and radiotherapy to ablate the bone marrow, followed by infusion of normal marrow from matched donors. There have been many problems with this approach but also there are now a number of long-term survivors, suggesting that, with further refinement, bone marrow transplantation, possibly combined with prior interferon therapy, may offer the possibility of cure for an increasing number of patients with CGL.

Chronic Lymphoid Leukaemia

As with CML the term chronic lymphoid leukaemia (CLL) is now recognised as embracing a number of different clinical entities. This discussion will be restricted to B-cell CLL, which makes up 95 per cent of all cases of CLL, and hairy-cell leukaemia which, although rare, is of interest because of recent developments in its treatment.

B-cell CLL

B-cell CLL has a peak incidence between 50 and 60 years and is rare below the age of 40 years. The disease is recognised as progressing through five clinical stages and the prognosis depends on the stage at the time of diagnosis (Table 15.2). Death is usually due to progressive bone marrow failure or impaired immunity but in 10 to 15 per cent of patients there is a terminal transition to either an acute lymphoma or acute leukaemia syndrome. Despite the often prolonged course of the disease, permanent cure of B-cell CLL is virtually unknown.

Treatment is related to the stage of the disease. For stage 0 no active therapy is indicated and in stages I and II local radiotherapy is given only if there are symptoms of pain or discomfort from enlarged nodes or spleno-megaly (in contrast to CML splenic irradiation has little or no effect on the systemic disease). Trials of various therapeutic approaches are currently

Table 15.2. Staging of chronic lymphoid leukaemia

Stage	Clinical features	Median survival (months)
0	Lymphocytosis confined to blood and bone marrow	120–180
I	Lymphocytosis with palpable lymphadenopathy	80–100
II	Lymphocytosis with hepatic or splenic enlargement	40–60
III	Lymphocytosis with anaemia	20–30
IV	Lymphocytosis with thrombocytopenia	15–30

underway in stage I and II B-cell CLL but it still remains to be proven that any form of active therapy in early disease actually increases survival. Systemic treatment is indicated in stage III and IV disease. The two drugs most commonly used are prednisone and chlorambucil. Prednisone is usually given initially, because of its lack of myelotoxicity, and chlorambucil is added subsequently. Treatment is usually continued until symptomatic relief is obtained or bone marrow failure controlled. Long-term maintenance therapy has no proven value and carries the risk of toxicity.

Combination chemotherapy is occasionally beneficial in resistant cases, with regimes such as COP (cyclophosphamide, vincristine and prednisone) or CHOP (COP plus doxorubicin). More recent developments in treatment include interferon administration and total body irradiation but the value of these approaches has still to be confirmed.

Hairy-cell leukaemia

Hairy-cell leukaemia accounts for only 2 per cent of the leukaemias and is predominantly a disease of middle age, affecting men four times more often than women. The most consistent clinical feature is splenomegaly. In the past splenectomy and chlorambucil administration have been the mainstays of treatment but it is now clear that interferon has a major effect in this disease and induces long-lasting complete remissions in some 90 per cent of patients. Whether the introduction of interferon will improve overall survival in this disease, which previously averaged 5 to 6 years, remains to be seen.

Hodgkin's Disease

The outlook for patients with Hodgkin's disease has improved dramatically over the past 25 years. In the early 1960s it was still considered an almost invariably fatal form of cancer, whereas today well over 50 per cent of patients will be completely cured. This change in prognosis has resulted from the introduction of improved treatment (with wide-field radiotherapy and combination chemotherapy) together with a recognition of the importance of accurately determining the stage of disease at the time of diagnosis in order to select the optimum therapy.

Once diagnosed, the disease is classified into one of four histological subtypes: lymphocyte predominant (5 to 10 per cent of cases, with a very good prognosis), nodular sclerosis (60 per cent of cases, with a good prognosis), mixed cellularity (30 per cent of cases, with a good prognosis) and lymphocyte depleted (5 to 10 per cent of cases, with a relatively poor prognosis). Staging is then carried out based on clinical examination, routine blood tests, bone marrow biopsy and CT scanning of the chest, abdomen and pelvis. The latter investigation has tended to displace lymphangiography and laporotomy which were previously essential parts of the staging procedure. The staging system used is shown in Table 15.3. The same system is used for the non-Hodgkin's lymphomas except that the subclassification into A and B categories is omitted.

Table 15.3.   Staging of Hodgkin's disease. Each stage is subdivided into A or B categories depending on the presence or absence of systemic symptoms. If weight loss of greater than 10 per cent, unexplained fever of 38°C or more, or night sweats are present the patient is in category B, if they are absent the patient is in category A.

Stage I
Involvement of a single group of lymph nodes or localised involvement of a single extralymphatic organ or site.

Stage II
Involvement of two or more groups of lymph nodes on the same side of the diaphragm, or localised involvement of a single extralymphatic organ or site and of one or more lymph node groups on the same side of the diaphragm.

Stage III
Involvement of lymph node groups on both sides of the diaphragm with or without localised involvement of a single extralymphatic organ or site and with or without splenic involvement.

Stage IV
Diffuse involvement of one or more extralymphatic organs or tissues with or without involvement of associated lymph nodes.

Studies in early stage disease carried out in the 1950s and 60s showed that local radiotherapy to involved lymph node groups invariably resulted in recurrence in adjacent glands and that, in order to achieve cure, regional treatment was necessary so that contiguous, apparently normal, lymph node groups were included in the radiation field. As a result wide-field radiotherapy was developed. This involves the irradiation of all lymphoid tissue on one or other side of the diaphragm. Thus, mantle fields cover the cervical, supraclavicular, axillary and mediastinal nodes whilst the inverted-Y technique includes para-aortic, iliac and inguinal nodes together with the spleen (Figure 15.1). The usual radiation dose is 35 to 40 Gray, given over 3 to 4 weeks. For some stages of disease total nodal irradiation is used with sequential treatment to mantle and inverted-Y fields.

Combination chemotherapy first made a major impact in the disease about 20 years ago when DeVita and his colleagues, at the National Cancer

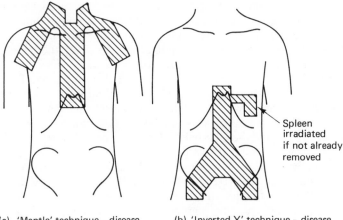

(a) 'Mantle' technique – disease   (b) 'Inverted Y' technique – disease
    confined above the diaphragm   confined below the diaphragm

Figure 15.1.   Wide field radiation for Hodgkin's disease.

Institute, introduced the MOPP regime, using four drugs (nitrogen mustard, vincristine [Oncovin], procarbazine and prednisolone) which had all previously been shown to have limited activity when used as single agents (De Vita V T et al, Annals of Internal Medicine, 73: 891–895, 1970). This regime, or variations of it, is still widely used today. (Modifications have included the substitution of chlorambucil for nitrogen mustard and vinblastine for vincristine, both intended to reduce toxicity.) Although this regime has completely changed the outlook in advanced Hodgkin's disease it is associated with the risk of second cancers in long-term survivors and also results in infertility in virtually all males and a significant proportion of females. In an attempt to reduce these hazards Bonadonna and his colleagues, in Milan, developed the ABVD (doxorubicin [Adriamycin], bleomycin, vinblastine and dacarbazine) regime in the mid-1970s (Bonadonna G et al, Cancer, 36: 252–259, 1975). This appears to have equivalent efficacy to MOPP in the control of Hodgkin's disease. It also reduces the risk of second malignancies and infertility but it is associated with more immediate toxicity, particularly severe nausea and vomiting, and there is an increased risk of late cardiopulmonary toxicity (due to bleomycin and doxorubicin). The relative merits of the two regimes as first-line therapies are still debated but, more importantly, the two combinations appear to be non-cross resistant and in recent years results have been further improved by giving alternating courses of MOPP and ABVD in advanced stages of the disease. When used alone, MOPP and ABVD are usually given for six courses, over about 6 months: when used as alternating regimes, a total of eight courses is the norm.

For stages IA, IB and IIA disease wide-field radiotherapy, with either mantle or inverted-Y fields as appropriate, is the treatment of choice. Some patients with stage IIA Hodgkin's disease, particularly those with nodular sclerosis, may present with bulky mediastinal node involvement. When this exceeds one third of the diameter of the lung fields, chemotherapy is indicated prior to irradiation. Either MOPP or ABVD are used but the number of courses is usually reduced to four. This combination of chemotherapy and radiation has also been recommended for stage IIA patients who have 3 or more node groups involved or who are over 40 years of age.

The optimum management of stage IIIA disease remains uncertain. Total nodal irradiation, chemotherapy plus total nodal irradiation and chemotherapy alone have all been used with no definite advantage emerging for any one approach. One fact that is now clear is that combining radiotherapy and chemotherapy significantly increases the risk of inducing second cancers. As a result there is a tendency to restrict treatment to one or other modality or to limit the use of radiotherapy after chemotherapy to local irradiation of sites of previous bulky disease. Stage IIB, IIIB and IVA and B disease are managed by chemotherapy, with increasing use of alternating drug schedules.

These various approaches to the management of Hodgkin's disease, together with their results, are summarised in Table 15.4.

Table 15.4.   Treatment and survival in Hodgkin's disease

Stage	Treatment	Complete response (per cent)	10-year survival (per cent)
IA, IB, IIA	Wide-field radiotherapy	90	85
IIA with bulky disease, age over 40 years, or 3 or more node groups involved	Chemotherapy plus radiotherapy	90	75
IIIA	Total nodal irradiation or chemotherapy or a combination of the two	90	80
IIB, IIIB, IVA, IVB	Chemotherapy	80	70

Non-Hodgkin's Lymphoma

The non-Hodgkin's lymphomas (NHL) are a diverse group of cancers and their precise classification has been an area of confusion for many years. By the early 1980s at least six different nomenclatures, based on histological appearance, were in use (Rappaport, Kiel, Lukes & Collins, WHO, British National Lymphoma Investigation and Dorfman classifications). In 1982, the National Cancer Institute published the results of a major survey based on a comparison of these various schemes and correlating microscopic appearance with clinical outcome (Rosenberg S A et al, Cancer, 49: 2112–2135, 1982). This resulted in a new classification, shown in Table 15.5, which defined NHLs in terms of their aggressiveness as either low-grade, intermediate grade or high-grade. In terms of practical management these three subgroups fall

Table 15.5.   Classification of non-Hodgkin's lymphoma

Histological classification	Cell of origin	Median survival (years)	Clinical course
Low-grade (34%)			
Malignant lymphoma, small cell lymphocytic (4%)		5.8	Indolent
Malignant lymphoma, follicular mainly small-cell cleaved (22%)	99% B-cell	7.2	Indolent
Malignant lymphoma, follicular mixed, small-cell cleaved and large cell (8%)		5.1	Indolent
Intermediate grade (38%)			
Malignant lymphoma, diffuse small-cell cleaved (7%)		3.4	Indolent
Malignant lymphoma, follicular mainly large cell (4%)	70% B-cell	3.0	Aggressive
Malignant lymphoma, diffuse mixed, small and large cell (7%)	20% T-cell	2.7	Aggressive
Malignant lymphoma, diffuse, large cell (20%)	5% Histiocytic	1.5	Aggressive
High-grade	5% Unclassified		
Malignant lymphoma, large cell, immunoblastic (8%)		1.3	Aggressive
Malignant lymphoma small non-cleaved cell		—	Aggressive
Malignant lymphoma, lymphoblastic (4%)		2.0	Aggressive
Miscellaneous			
Includes mycosis fungoides, Sezary syndrome, hairy-cell leukaemia	Mainly B-cell	—	Variable

into three separate categories with different therapeutic approaches being required for the more indolent lymphomas, the more aggressive lymphomas and lymphoblastic lymphoma (see Table 15.6).

Paradoxically, although overall survival times are longer in indolent NHL, these tumours are more frequently disseminated at presentation and, when widespread, they are rarely, if ever, cured. By contrast, advances in treatment over the last 10 to 15 years have resulted in complete regressions of 3 to 5 years in well over 50 per cent of patients with disseminated aggressive NHL, suggesting that permanent cure may be possible in a significant proportion of these cases.

As with Hodgkin's disease, the treatment of NHL depends on the stage of the disease. Approximately 20 per cent of indolent tumours and 40 per cent of aggressive NHL will be stage I or II at presentation. For these cancers, local radiotherapy, to a dose of 40 Gray over 4 weeks, is the treatment of choice. In contrast to Hodgkin's disease there is no need for wide-field irradiation, only the involved glands, or organ, and immediately adjacent nodes being

Table 15.6.   Treatment and survival in non-Hodgkin's lymphoma (NHL)

Tumour	Treatment	Complete response rate (per cent)	5-year survival (per cent)
Indolent NHL			
Stage I/II	Radiotherapy	90	75
Stage III/IV	No treatment, low dose steroids and/or low dose cytotoxic drugs	90	50
Aggressive NHL			
Stage I	Radiotherapy	90	80
Stage II	Radiotherapy	80	70
Stage III/IV	Combination cytotoxic chemotherapy	70	60

included in the treatment volume. Long-term survival, with a good chance of permanent cure, is possible in more than 50 per cent of patients (Table 15.6).

For patients with disseminated indolent NHL (stages III and IV) it is important to realise that although permanent cure is seldom, if ever, achieved, the disease usually runs a very protracted course, with little or no effect on the general health of the patient for many years. Therefore, particularly in elderly patients, active treatment is only indicated when troublesome symptoms develop. First-line therapy in this situation is either oral prednisolone or low-dose oral cytotoxic therapy with drugs such as chlorambucil, cyclophosphamide or the nitrosoureas. Sometimes, alkylating agents and corticosteroids are combined but there is no evidence that this, or any more aggressive drug combination, improves the results of treatment. Overall, some 90 per cent of patients will respond to these measures and in over 60 per cent there will be complete disappearance of disease. Ultimately, however, relapse is almost inevitable and although further courses of single-agent therapy may induce another remission the disease will eventually become resistant to such treatment. At this stage a variety of therapeutic options is available, including total lymphoid or whole-body irradiation, combination chemotherapy (with schedules similar to those used for aggressive NHL) and interferon. Although further remissions may be achieved as a result of these measures the duration of response is usually far less than that seen with the initial treatment. The relative merits of the various second-line treatments are still being determined in current clinical trials and, as yet, no uniform treatment policy exists.

For those with advanced aggressive NHL, combination chemotherapy forms the mainstay of treatment. Four- or five-drug regimens, introduced in the early 1970s, produced complete responses in about 50 per cent of patients, with more than half of the responders surviving to 5 years. Two of the most widely used combinations were CHOP (cyclophosphamide, doxorubicin, vincristine and prednisone) and BACOP (bleomycin, doxorubicin, cyclophosphamide, vincristine and prednisone). Building on this initial success, more recent programmes have either increased the number of drugs in the combination (adding such agents as methotrexate, a nitrosourea or etoposide) or have used alternating courses of different agents. These moves have increased response rates to over 70 per cent with the majority of responses lasting over 5 years, suggesting that many of the patients might be permanently cured. The precise drug combinations and dose schedules used are being constantly refined and there is every reason to suppose that a further improvement in response rates and survival will be seen over the next few years.

Lymphoblastic NHL is a very aggressive disease, most commonly seen in children and adolescents. In contrast to the other high-grade lymphomas, it is treated in a similar way to acute lymphoblastic leukaemia, although the results of treatment are less encouraging than those seen in ALL.

Polycythaemia Vera

Polycythaemia is an overproduction of the red blood cells leading to an increase in total red cell volume. It is often seen as a physiological response in chronic anoxic conditions, such as emphysema and cyanotic heart disease, but may also occur as a primary cancer of the bone marrow resulting in uncontrolled red cell production which is ultimately fatal. This latter condition is referred to as polycythaemia vera to distinguish it from physiological polycythaemia. The disease runs a very protracted course and even in untreated patients the median survival is seven years.

Three methods of treatment are available: venesection (simply withdrawing approximately 500ml of blood at regular intervals to regulate the total red cell volume); radiotherapy (with the injection of radioactive phosphorus) and chemotherapy (traditionally using single drug therapy with an alkylating agent such as busulphan, chlorambucil or melphalan).

Long-term clinical trials have now compared these three approaches and the results show that up to 7 years the survival figures are similar but thereafter survival declines quite rapidly in those given chemotherapy. This is due to the development of second malignancies and, in some series, as many as 50 per cent of patients given alkylating agents have died of second cancers. There is also an increased risk of second tumours following radioactive phosphorus administration but these tumours occur less often and later than those seen after chlorambucil or busulphan.

As a result of these findings there has been increasing interest in the use of hydroxyurea, which is not an alkylating agent, as an alternative form of chemotherapy. This drug certainly produces responses in the great majority of patients but, although there is little evidence of carcinogenicity as yet, it is still too early to be certain of the long-term consequences of treatment. Overall, average survival times with venesection and radioactive phosphorus are in excess of 10 years and it remains to be seen whether hydroxyurea can improve on these results.

Multiple Myeloma

Multiple myeloma is a cancer of the plasma cells within the bone marrow. It is a relatively uncommon condition characterised by the appearance of excessive numbers of abnormal plasma cells within the bone marrow, bone destruction and the production of abnormal plasma proteins.

In the early 1960s, alkylating agents were found to be of value in this disease and good results were obtained with both melphalan and cyclophosphamide, when used as single agents. In 1971, these two agents were compared in a Medical Research Council trial and found to be equally effective. It was subsequently shown that combining prednisone with melphalan increases response rates but that overall survival was not increased. About 50 per cent of patients will gain a remission with these drugs but the remissions are almost always partial rather than complete and cure is virtually unknown.

Patients who have myeloma may be divided into a poor risk group, who have anaemia or evidence of renal failure or hypercalcaemia, or a good risk group with none of these features. Untreated, the overall survival is about seven months but the use of alkylating agents, with or without steroids, has increased life expectancy in good risk patients to over four years and in the poor risk group to about two years. Recent attempts to try and improve these figures have involved a wide range of different combination chemotherapy schedules but although response rates have been increased there is no convincing evidence of enhanced survival. Interferons have some activity in myeloma and their role is currently being evaluated; certainly they are not superior to alkyating agent therapy, but whether they may improve survival if combined with conventional cytotoxics remains to be seen. Other new approaches to treatment currently being assessed include wide-field radiotherapy and bone marrow transplantation.

Symptomatic and supportive therapy is of great importance in patients with myeloma and radiotherapy remains the treatment of choice for bone pain due to myeloma deposits.

Chapter 16

Solid Tumours

Lung Cancer

The results of treatment in lung cancer depend on three main factors: the histological type of the tumour, the stage of disease and the general condition of the patient. From a therapeutic viewpoint the various histological types of lung cancer can be divided into two main groups: small cell carcinomas (also called oat-cell carcinomas), which make up about 20 per cent of cases, and non-small cell cancers, which form the remaining 80 per cent of bronchogenic carcinomas, including squamous cell carcinomas, adenocarcinomas and large cell cancers. The management of these two forms of lung cancer differs considerably.

Small Cell Lung Cancer

The approach to treatment, and its results, depend on the stage of the disease at the time of diagnosis. At presentation about 30 per cent of patients have limited stage disease, with tumour apparently confined to one hemithorax, whilst the remaining 70 per cent will have extensive disease, with widespread lung involvement or distant metastases. Even in those patients who appear to have limited disease it is recognised that micrometastases are invariably present and localised treatment alone will therefore be inadequate. Untreated small cell lung cancer is an aggressive disease with a median survival of only 2 to 3 months but the tumour is chemosensitive and drug treatment forms the cornerstone of management. A variety of drugs have activity in this condition, but two combinations have come to the forefront in recent years: these are vincristine, doxorubicin and cyclophosphamide (VAC) and cisplatinum plus etoposide.

Vigorous chemotherapy, usually with alternating courses of VAC and cisplatinum and etoposide given over 4 to 6 months, produces regressions in about 90 per cent of patients with limited stage disease, about half of these being complete responses. The median survival is increased from about 3 to

14 months with some 10 per cent of patients alive and disease free at two years. Unfortunately, late relapses still occur and by five years survival is reduced to about 5 per cent but, nonetheless, it is still likely that a small percentage of patients are now being cured of this previously uniformly fatal condition as a result of chemotherapy.

Efforts are now being made to increase the proportion of long-term survivors. Intensifying chemotherapy and/or giving sustained maintenance therapy do not appear beneficial. The use of radiotherapy or surgery as adjuvants to chemotherapy, with the intention of preventing local relapse in the chest, is currently being explored but, although it is clear that such procedures reduce the risk of local recurrence from around 70 per cent to less than 30 per cent, their effect on survival is uncertain.

Similarly, prophylactic brain irradiation reduces the incidence of cerebral secondaries from 40 per cent to less than 10 per cent but, once again, the impact of this on survival is not clear and there are anxieties about the late effects of such treatment in those patients who survive beyond 2 years.

For those patients who have extensive disease at the time of diagnosis there is, as yet, no prospect of cure and treatment is, therefore, generally less intensive. The use of either VAC or cisplatinum plus etoposide will bring about remissions in 60 to 80 per cent of patients with about 25 per cent of these being complete responses. Median survival times are increased by treatment but only from about 1.5 months to 8 months.

Non-small Cell Lung Cancer

Localised tumours lying in the periphery of the lung or more than 2cm from the carina are best treated by surgery or radical radiotherapy. Depending on the precise location and extent of disease 5-year survivals of 30 to 60 per cent may be expected and many of these patients will be cured, although a significant minority will develop second bronchogenic cancers. Unfortunately, however, the great majority of patients have extensive disease at the time of presentation, rendering them ineligible for radical local therapy. Radiation remains an effective form of palliation for these patients, relieving symptoms such as dyspnoea, cough, haemoptysis, chest pain and superior vena cava obstruction in more than 60 per cent of cases. There is no evidence, however, that such treatment increases survival.

Many cytotoxic agents have been evaluated in non-small cell lung cancer but only four have demonstrated significant activity, with response rates of about 20 per cent when given as single agents: these are cisplatinum, ifosfamide, mitomycin-C and vindesine. Various combinations of these agents have been used and response rates as high as 50 per cent have been claimed. At present, however, there is no evidence that the use of chemotherapy increases median survival beyond the 4 to 5 months that is seen when treatment is confined to purely palliative measures. There is, therefore little justification for the use of routine cytotoxic therapy in this condition and such treatment should be restricted to controlled clinical trials evaluating new therapeutic approaches.

Carcinoma of the Breast

Considerable space is devoted to breast cancer in this chapter, partly because it is the commonest cancer to affect women (about 1 in 15 women will develop breast cancer) and also because it is highly responsive to systemic therapy and even in its advanced stages often runs a protracted course over many years. For these reasons breast cancer often accounts for more than half the workload of departments devoted to the chemotherapy of solid tumours.

Although carcinoma of the breast is so common, with some 21,000 new cases registered each year in England and Wales, there is no universal agreement on the best approach to its management, a situation which is, in part, due to the multiplicity of treatment options available and the constant development of new ways of integrating these into an overall treatment strategy. Furthermore, although the disease is clearly very sensitive to systemic therapy, the precise impact of such therapy on overall survival remains uncertain. The following summary is an attempt to highlight some of the current issues and policies in the management of breast cancer.

Early Breast Cancer

Early breast cancer is defined as a mobile tumour within the breast (not fixed either to the overlying skin or underlying muscle), with or without ipsilateral axillary node metastases. For many years the treatment of this condition relied on purely local treatment – a mastectomy, either alone or combined with post-operative irradiation. In the last 10 years there has been a growing realisation that for most patients very limited surgery, simply removing the primary cancer in the breast with a small margin of normal tissue (a lumpectomy) combined with post-operative radiotherapy to the breast and axillary region gives equivalent results to the more radical, and mutilating, surgical procedures of the past. This change in local therapy has obvious psychological and cosmetic advantages but has no influence on overall survival rates.

The reason for this lack of improvement is the natural history of the disease. Patients with breast cancer do not die from their local disease but from distant metastases, and in many women these metastases, although not clinically apparent, are present at the time of their initial treatment. However good the technique, surgery and radiotherapy are only local treatments and will not control distant secondaries so even if the primary growth is completely eradicated these patients will still die from breast cancer.

The likelihood of occult metastases being present correlates well with the clinical stage of the disease. Patients who have a freely mobile lump in the breast with no axillary spread have a more than 70 per cent chance of being alive and disease-free 5 years after primary treatment. If there are one to three axillary nodes involved with tumour this figure falls to 60 per cent and if more than three glands contain metastases there is a further reduction to less than 40 per cent.

The very good remissions seen following cytotoxic therapy in women with advanced breast cancer led a number of clinicians, in the mid 1970s, to assess the drugs as adjuvant therapy in women who underwent initial surgery but who were found to have axillary metastases and hence a high risk of harbouring distant micrometastases. The early results of these studies indicated a considerable reduction in relapse rates for those who received the drugs, although it was not clear whether this would translate into improved survival. The optimism generated by these findings was tempered by worries about the toxicity of chemotherapy, especially as a significant proportion of the women treated would already have been cured by the initial surgery and were, therefore, being needlessly exposed to the short-term discomfort and, largely unknown, long-term hazards of cytotoxic administration. At this time, tamoxifen had recently become available and was rapidly being recognised as a major agent in the management of advanced disease. It was soon introduced into the adjuvant setting, as a gentler alternative to cytotoxics. Five- to ten-year follow-up data are now available from a number of large adjuvant studies and although it is still too early to make absolute judgements a number of interim observations may be made:

1. A number of studies indicate an increased time to relapse in women receiving adjuvant chemotherapy compared to those who do not. This increase in relapse-free survival is of very doubtful significance, as those women who have not had previous drug treatment may do so on relapse and gain a subsequent remission, whereas those who have already had adjuvant chemotherapy will, if they relapse, have to rely on second-line drug treatment with a reduced chance of response. Thus the overall survival rate, rather than disease-free survival, is the definitive measure of the value of adjuvant therapy.

2. Cytotoxic therapy definitely increases absolute survival in premenopausal women who have 1 to 3 axillary nodes involved with tumour, with about 70 per cent of women who received chemotherapy being alive at 10 years compared to only 50 per cent of those who did not. Although relapse-free survival is increased, there is no evidence of enhancement of overall survival in those women with four or more nodes involved.

3. Most adjuvant cytotoxic regimes have been based on the combination of cyclophosphamide, methotrexate and 5-fluorouracil, although single agent melphalan has also been used quite extensively. There is no agreement, as yet, on the optimum drug combination in this situation and the question of drug dose remains controversial. There is increasing agreement that cytotoxic therapy should begin as soon as possible after initial surgery and that prolonging treatment beyond six months probably does not improve the results and is, therefore, unnecessary.

4. Virtually all women who undergo adjuvant cytotoxic therapy develop amenorrhoea. The extent to which cytotoxic therapy may actually be achieving its effect by a secondary hormonal mechanism - as a result of ovarian suppression - rather than a direct cytotoxic action, remains unclear.

5. There is no evidence of enhanced survival in post-menopausal patients with cytotoxic therapy.

6. Results from adjuvant studies using tamoxifen are now showing an overall survival advantage for patients in both pre- and post-menopausal age groups. The increase is not as great as that seen in premenopausal women given cytotoxic therapy but still equates with about a 15 to 20 per cent increase in survival at 5 years. Surprisingly, although the benefit is greater for women whose tumours are oestrogen receptor-positive there is still a beneficial effect in those whose lesions are receptor-negative.

7. A dose of 20mg once daily is sufficient to achieve these results but the optimum duration of tamoxifen therapy remains uncertain. It has usually been given for at least two years and, in contrast to cytotoxic therapy, there is some theoretical evidence suggesting that continuing treatment indefinitely may be beneficial.

Advanced Breast Cancer

The term advanced breast cancer embraces both patients who present with advanced disease (tumours which are fixed either to the skin overlying, or the muscle underlying, the breast, which are invariably associated with occult distant metastases, or those who have overt disease outside the breast and axilla at the time of diagnosis) and those who develop local recurrence or distant metastases following initial treatment for early lesions. Although radiotherapy may be invaluable for relief of local symptoms (such as bone pain) control of the disease overall at this stage requires a systemic treatment. In the past, those women presenting *de novo* with advanced disease and those relapsing after primary treatment have been managed in a similar way but the increasing use of adjuvant drug therapy has complicated the treatment of the latter group by reducing the therapeutic options available.

There are numerous systemic treatments available for advanced breast cancer and the first choice to be made is whether to use endocrine or cytotoxic therapy. The principal factors influencing this decision are the rate of progress of the disease, the site of metastases and the hormone receptor status of the tumour. Responses to endocrine therapy usually take several months to become apparent whereas patients who are going to respond to cytotoxics start to show an improvement within 3 to 4 weeks of starting treatment. Thus, cytotoxic chemotherapy is indicated as first-line therapy for the relatively small group of women who have rapidly progressive disease. Liver metastases tend to be less sensitive to hormonal manoeuvres than secondaries at other sites (with the exception of cerebral metastases for which a combination of dexamethasone and whole-brain irradiation is usually prescribed) and many clinicians regard hepatic involvement as a definite indication for cytotoxic treatment. If, however, the tumour is very slow growing an initial trial of hormonal therapy is still justified. Patients whose tumours are hormone receptor-positive have a far greater chance of responding to endocrine treatment than those whose tumours are receptor-negative (see Chapter 11) and, unless the disease is progressing very rapidly, one would always use hormonal therapies initially for these women. Somewhere, between 10 and 20 per cent of receptor-negative tumours will, however, still respond to endocrine treatment, so for those women whose lesions are receptor-negative, and for those in whom the receptor status is not known, an initial trial of hormone treatment is still justified, provided that the disease is relatively slow growing.

Although overall response rates are higher with cytotoxic chemotherapy than with endocrine treatment, prospective studies have shown that, with the possible exception of those women with very aggressive, fast growing tumours, overall survival is not influenced by the order in which the two treatments are given and so less toxic endocrine therapy is generally preferred by most oncologists as the first approach to treatment. Similarly, prospective clinical trials have demonstrated that giving cytotoxic and hormonal therapy simultaneously increases the initial response rate but does not increase survival and so most clinicians adopt a sequential approach to management rather than combining the two modalities.

Endocrine Therapy

By the early 1970s the pattern of endocrine treatment for advanced breast cancer had become reasonably uniform with premenopausal patients being treated by ovarian ablation (either oophorectomy or a radiation-induced menopause) and post-menopausal women receiving additive therapy with either oestrogens or androgens. For those who relapsed after an initial response the choice lay between the ablative procedures of either adrenalectomy or hypophysectomy and additive treatment with low-dose progestogens or corticosteroids.

The introduction of tamoxifen in the early 1970s changed this picture, for although its response rate (30 to 35 per cent) and median duration of response (18 to 24 months) were similar to those seen with oestrogens and androgens, tamoxifen caused significantly less toxicity than these agents in terms of both the incidence and the severity of side effects. It therefore soon became accepted as the first-line endocrine treatment for post-menopausal women. Its role in premenopausal patients, however, still remains uncertain. The limited number of prospective evaluations which have been carried out suggest that the efficacy of tamoxifen is equivalent to that of ovarian ablation, but many clinicans still prefer the latter treatment. The fact that about two thirds of women continue to menstruate whilst taking tamoxifen (although approximately half of these will have scanty and irregular periods) has raised the possibility that combining tamoxifen and ovarian ablation may enhance the results. Tamoxifen has, however, been combined with other endocrine therapies with no improvement in overall survival and so the chances of a benefit from this approach are small.

Aminoglutethimide, developed in the mid-1970s, and high-dose progestogen therapy, introduced in the early 1980s, both offer response rates and response durations similar to those seen with tamoxifen, but their greater toxicity has prevented them from displacing it as first-line therapy. These drugs have, however, displaced oestrogens, androgens and adrenal or pituitary ablation as second-line therapies. Fifty per cent of those patients who respond initially to tamoxifen and then relapse will gain a further remission with second-line endocrine therapy and, of those women who experience no benefit from tamoxifen, some 20 per cent will respond to other hormonal agents. Second-line therapy is, therefore, an important aspect of endocrine treatment in advanced breast cancer and the results of high-dose medroxy-progesterone acetate and aminoglutethimide in this situation have recently been formally compared in a prospective trial (Canney P A et al, Journal of the National Cancer Institute, 1988, 80: 147–151). Both agents gave equivalent responses to treatment and a further 20 per cent of patients showing an objective response to treatment and a further 20 per cent benefiting from stabilisation of previously progressive disease, the remissions lasting for an average of about twelve months. Furthermore, a number of patients who relapsed then gained another remission by switching to the alternative drug, indicating that even third-line endocrine therapy is still effective for some patients.

One interesting phenomenon in additive endocrine therapy is that of the withdrawal response. In the past, it was well recognised that about 20 per cent of patients who gained a remission with oestrogen therapy would, on relapse, gain a further benefit simply from withdrawal of the drug with no additional therapy. The same pattern has now been clearly documented with tamoxifen and it is apparent that on relapse about 15 per cent of women will go into remission, often for many months, simply as a result of stopping the drug.

Cytotoxic Therapy

Many cytotoxic drugs produce response rates of 20 to 40 per cent when used as single agents in advanced breast cancer. It is now well-established that this response rate may be further increased by combining agents, although it is still a matter of debate as to whether this actually increases overall survival. During the 1970s numerous combination regimes were devised and objective responses were claimed in anything from 20 to 100 per cent of patients. It is now clear that this enormous variation had more to do with variable patient selection and dubious response criteria than with differences in drug efficacy. Overall, combination cytotoxic therapy produces objective response in 50 to 60 per cent of patients (approximately double the response rate of endocrine therapy) but the responses are generally shorter than those seen with hormonal treatment, lasting six to nine months on average. Despite numerous claims to the contrary, no single regime has established itself as the optimum therapy in this indication. Most schedules are built round combinations of cyclophospha-mide, methotrexate and 5-fluorouracil or use doxorubicin (the most active single agent in advanced breast cancer) combined with one or more drugs, most often vincristine.

The realisation in the mid 1980s that a plateau in therapeutic results from cytotoxic therapy had been reached has led to two different responses. On the one hand, it has been argued that if aggressive regimes do no better than gentler treatments then efforts should be concentrated on developing cyto-toxic schedules which maintain efficacy but keep toxicity to a minimum. This has resulted in an increased emphasis on quality of life in this group of patients and a reversion to single agent therapy in many cases, using newer, less toxic agents, such as mitozantrone and epirubicin. The alternative view has been that the full potential of cytotoxic therapy has not been realised simply because treatment was not adequate and that more aggressive therapy, with particular attention to dose intensity (see Chapter 4) is needed to improve results. The relationship between drug dose and response in advanced breast cancer is still debated, as are issues such as the optimum duration of cytotoxic treatment and the value of using alternating non-cross resistant regimes. Thus, although over the years more patients with advanced breast cancer have received cytotoxic therapy than in any other disease, the optimum schedule for and precise value of such treatment remain to be determined.

Despite these uncertainties, it is clear that although the median survival for women with advanced breast cancer is only of the order of two years a substantial number of patients, particularly those who are highly hormone-responsive may survive for many years, with an excellent quality of life, as a result of carefully sequenced endocrine and cytotoxic therapy.

Gastrointestinal Cancer

The great majority of gastrointestinal cancers are adenocarcinomas arising from the stomach, pancreas or large bowel. Surgery is the primary treatment for gastrointestinal adenocarcinomas, with radiotherapy and cytotoxic therapy usually being reserved for the palliation of advanced or inoperable disease. Recently, however, a number of studies have suggested that post-operative irradiation following resection of rectal carcinomas may reduce local recurrence rates although whether this improves overall survival remains to be determined.

Considerable pessimism surrounds the use of chemotherapy in these tumours. For many years 5-fluorouracil has been considered the agent of choice for gastrointestinal adenocarcinoma. Attempts to improve the results of treatment have concentrated largely on different techniques of administration and variation of the dose schedule of 5-fluorouracil rather than exploring other drugs. 5-Fluorouracil has been given orally, by prolonged intravenous infusion, intra-arterially into the hepatic artery or aorta (for patients with liver metastases) or intraluminally into the rectum. None of these regimes has improved on the results of weekly intravenous injection, following an initial 4 to 6 day loading dose, given intravenously. Such treatment has led to overall response rates of 20 to 30 per cent, although there is no evidence that survival is improved.

Other drugs which have shown activity in gastrointestinal adenocarcinomas include mitomycin-C, the nitrosoureas, doxorubicin (in gastric and pancreatic tumours) and melphalan (in large bowel cancers). None of these has proved superior to 5-fluorouracil but a number of combination regimes have been devised, based on these agents: FAM (5-fluorouracil, doxorubicin and mitomycin-C) has been widely used in gastric and pancreatic cancers whilst

MOF (methyl-CCNU, vincristine and 5-fluorouracil) has been employed for rectal and colonic lesions. Although response rates are modestly increased with such regimes there is no clear evidence that they actually enhance survival.

In recent years, there have been a number of studies evaluating adjuvant therapy with cytotoxic drugs in gastric and rectal carcinoma. The results are difficult to interpret as, although most trials have proved negative, there have been isolated studies where marginally improved survival rates have been claimed. Certainly these data are not sufficient to recommend routine use of adjuvant chemotherapy after surgery for these tumours but further clinical trials to clarify the situation are justified. One form of adjuvant chemotherapy which is attracting considerable interest at present is liver perfusion, with 5-fluorouracil being administered through the portal vein, following resection of large bowel carcinomas. There is some evidence that this technique reduces the likelihood of hepatic metastases appearing and definitive clinical trials evaluating this approach are currently in progress.

Two uncommon gastrointestinal cancers should also be mentioned: squamous cell carcinoma of the anal canal and malignant carcinoid tumour. In the past, anal cancers have been treated surgically, with an abdomino-perineal resection, or, occasionally, by local radiotherapy. Irradiation relied on the implantation of radioactive sources, such as caesium or radium needles, directly into the tumour and only a small proportion of anal carcinomas were suitable for such treatment. A number of recent reports have suggested that giving 5-fluorouracil and mitomycin-C concurrently with radical external beam radiotherapy offers cure rates equivalent to those seen with surgery, thus saving patients a major operation and a permanent colostomy. The relative rarity of squamous cell carcinomas of the anal canal means that comparative randomised trials are difficult to organise, but several such studies are now in progress, seeking to confirm the role of chemotherapy in these tumours. Malignant carcinoid tumours are even less common than anal carcinomas and have generally proved resistant to cytotoxic drugs, but there is increasing evidence that they may be sensitive to interferons and this possibility is being actively explored at the present time.

Genitourinary Cancer

Carcinoma of the Prostate

This is predominantly a tumour of the elderly and is the commonest cancer in men over 65 years of age. The tumour often lies dormant within the prostate gland, causing no symptoms, and is only discovered as an incidental finding at post-mortem. Of those cancers presenting clinically the majority have already metastasised to the bones by the time of diagnosis. For the minority of localised lesions the treatment is either radical prostatectomy or radiotherapy. The results of these two procedures are similar with some 80 per cent of men whose tumours are confined to the prostate surviving 5 years after treatment: if the tumour is infiltrating the tissues immediately surrounding the gland this figure falls to 65 per cent.

In metastatic disease androgen suppression will lead to a remission in 80 per cent of patients with an average duration of response of 18 to 24 months. Despite this high response rate there is no clear evidence that treatment actually increases survival and so it is usual to delay the introduction of active therapy until symptoms develop. In the past orchidectomy or stilboestrol administration have formed the mainstay of treatment for metastatic disease. Both treatments give similar results, with response in some 80 per cent of men. Orchidectomy, however, although relatively free of side effects, is psychologically unacceptable to some patients whilst stilboestrol, at doses of 3 to 5 mg per day, is associated with a considerably increased risk of serious, and potentially fatal, cardiovascular symptoms. This risk is reduced with lower doses of the drug but at these levels the degree of androgen suppression is unpredictable.

New drugs have been developed to try and overcome these problems and both anti-androgens (cyproterone acetate and flutamide) and luteinising hormone releasing hormone (LHRH) analogues (buserilin and goserilin) have been evaluated. These drugs appear to offer response rates and remission durations similar to, but no better than, those seen with stilboestrol but offer the advantage of reduced toxicity (although they are considerably more expensive). It has been claimed that total androgen blockade, achieved by combining cyproterone and an LHRH analogue, improves the response rate but this remains to be substantiated and certainly previous combined hormonal therapies in prostatic cancer (for example oestrogen plus orchidectomy) have not shown any advantage over single modality treatment.

For patients who relapse after initial hormone therapy, or who fail to respond to such therapy, the outlook is poor with a median survival of only about 6 months. Second-line endocrine therapies seldom achieve a response and cytotoxic drugs have little or no activity in this tumour. Management is essentially symptomatic and radiotherapy is often an excellent means of relieving the pain from bone secondaries in these patients.

Carcinoma of the Kidney

The majority of kidney tumours in adults are adenocarcinomas arising in the renal cortex. The treatment of choice is surgical excision, with the addition of post-operative radiotherapy if there is any local extension of disease. In resectable cases, the five-year survival approaches 50 per cent but for the remainder the outlook is poor.

Cytotoxic therapy is of little or no value in metastatic disease. In the past, progestins have been used and response rates of 10 to 20 per cent have been claimed in some series. One of the difficulties in assessing the significance of such a low rate of remission is the fact that renal cell carcinoma may occasionally regress spontaneously for many months. The true incidence of such spontaneous remissions is uncertain but figures as high as 20 per cent have been suggested. If these figures are genuine then the active role of progestins in controlling metastases becomes highly questionable.

More recently, interferons have been shown to have activity in advanced renal cell carcinoma. The lungs are the commonest site of spread and somewhere between 25 and 40 per cent of patients with pulmonary secondaries will gain a response, which may last many months, from interferon therapy. Those whose metastatic disease is predominantly at other sites show only occasional responses and the value of interferons in such cases is doubtful.

Carcinoma of the Bladder

The role of intravesical chemotherapy in early, superficial bladder cancer has been discussed in Chapter 8.

For those tumours which are infiltrating into the muscle of the bladder wall at the time of presentation radiotherapy or radical cystectomy or a combination of the two are the usual approaches to treatment. Average five-year survival figures following such therapy are slightly less than 50 per cent. In the past, chemotherapy has been reserved for patients who relapse after primary treatment and for the 5 per cent who present with metastatic disease. Until recently, the results of drug treatment have been generally disappointing but in the last 10 years a number of studies have indicated that this situation may be changing.

It is now clear that methotrexate and cisplatinum are the two most active agents against transitional cell bladder carcinoma. Used singly, they give response rates of about 30 per cent in advanced disease, with some 5 per cent of remissions being complete. When used together, the response rate rises to between 50 and 70 per cent with complete responses increasing to 20 to 40 per cent. Although it is clear that those patients who respond to chemotherapy live longer than the non-responders, it is still uncertain whether these remissions are actually increasing overall survival in patients with advanced bladder cancer. Other agents which have activity in these tumours are doxorubicin, vincristine, vinblastine and mitomycin-C, but whether the addition of these to cisplatinum and methotrexate will further enhance response figures is not yet determined.

This increase in response in metastatic or relapsed disease has led to interest in exploring the adjuvant role of chemotherapy in those tumours with muscle penetration but no obvious metastatic spread. In particular, the role of neo-adjuvant treatment with cisplatinum and methotrexate, either alone or in combination, is being actively explored in a number of clinical trials. Early results showed an initial increase in two-year survival figures but longer follow-up suggests this benefit may not be sustained: the true value of neo-adjuvant therapy in transitional cell carcinoma of the bladder therefore remains to be determined.

Testicular Cancer

Although they account for only 1 per cent of cancers in men, testicular tumours are of great importance, partly because of the dramatic improvements in the results of treatment over the last 10 to 15 years and partly because they are the commonest solid tumour in those aged between 15 and 35 years.

Malignant testicular tumours arise from the spermatogonia and are therefore often referred to as germ-cell tumours. They are classified as either seminomas or teratomas. Seminomas account for about one third of cases: the remainder are either teratomas or mixed seminomas and teratomas, the latter being treated as teratomas although carrying a slightly more favourable prognosis. A significant proportion of teratomas produce the serum markers β-human chorionic gonadotrophin or α-fetaprotein, which can be serially measured to monitor the response to treatment.

Historically, the pattern of management was similar for both seminomas and teratomas: most patients appeared to have disease confined to the testis at the time of presentation and so orchidectomy was performed, but because it was recognised that there was often occult, microscopic, spread to the para-aortic nodes either adjuvant abdominal radiotherapy (favoured in the UK) or radical retroperitoneal lymph node dissection (favoured in the USA) were usually carried out. Chemotherapy was reserved for relapse, which was uncommon in seminomas but frequent, and invariably fatal, in teratomas.

Improvements in staging procedures now mean that more than 60 per cent of men with teratomas are identified as having tumour which has spread beyond the testis at the time of diagnosis. Improvements in chemotherapy mean that even those with widespread disease have a high chance of cure.

Until the early 1970s the results of chemotherapy for teratoma were disappointing but, at that time, the combination of vinblastine and bleomycin began to produce substantial numbers of long-term survivors in men with recurrent disease. The addition of cisplatinum to this regime in the late 1970s has boosted the long-term survival rate to over 80 per cent in those presenting with metastatic disease. More recently, etoposide has also been shown to have activity in this tumour and has been substituted for vinblastine with a consequent reduction in toxicity. Thus, for patients with widespread disease, the standard policy is 4 to 6 courses of chemotherapy. As a result of this about 70 per cent will go into complete, long-term remission and a further 10 to 20 per cent will have residual disease which is resectable and will achieve long-term remission and probable cure following surgery. Thus five-year survival rates in excess of 80 per cent are now being consistently achieved, whereas in 1970 the figure was less than 10 per cent.

This success in widespread disease has influenced the management of the earlier stages of teratoma. For those who have spread restricted to the retroperitoneal nodes three options are available, each giving virtually 100 per cent cure rates: chemotherapy alone, surgery (lymph node dissection) plus chemotherapy if relapse occurs or radiotherapy followed by chemotherapy if relapse occurs. Increasingly the move is towards chemotherapy alone, especially as there are indications that fewer courses of treatment may be needed than in advanced disease. For those patients whose tumour appears to be confined to the testis and whose serum markers return to normal following orchidectomy, there is a growing tendency to discard adjuvant retroperitoneal node dissection or irradiation in favour of careful follow-up alone, giving chemotherapy to the 20 to 30 per cent who ultimately relapse.

Seminomas are less aggressive than teratomas. The traditional approach of orchidectomy and post-operative retroperitoneal node irradiation cures the great majority of patients and has not been seriously questioned. For those patients who do relapse, or who present with widespread disease, single agent cisplatinum is highly effective and potentially curative.

Gynaecological Cancer

Carcinoma of the Cervix

The emphasis in the management of carcinoma of the cervix over the last 25 years has been on early diagnosis and, in Britain, this has resulted in a modest increase in cure rates, but the overall five-year survival is still only of the order of 55 per cent. Primary treatment relies on radiotherapy, or surgery, or a combination of the two. In the past, the results of chemotherapy for those patients who relapse have been disappointing. By the early 1980s it was established that a number of drugs used as single agents produced responses of a few months in 15 to 20 per cent of patients: these drugs included doxorubicin, methotrexate and bleomycin. Subsequently, two agents, cisplatinum and ifosfamide, have shown a higher level of activity with response rates of the order of 30 per cent.

Based on these results a number of combination regimes have been explored in metastatic cervical carcinoma in recent years. Most of these have failed to produce response rates greater than 30 per cent and, when responses have been seen, their median duration has only been about 3 to 4 months. Currently, however, the combinations of bleomycin plus cisplatinum and bleomycin, cisplatinum plus ifosfamide are consistently producing responses in over 50 per cent of patients and appear to represent a genuine advance in treatment. Encouraged by these results a number of oncologists are now exploring the value of these regimes as neo-adjuvant therapies for those women with tumour extending outside the cervix but still, clinically, confined to the pelvis.

Carcinoma of the Endometrium

About 75 per cent of endometrial adenocarcinomas are confined to the uterine body at the time of diagnosis. Surgery is the cornerstone of treatment for such tumours and results in a five-year survival of around 70 per cent. Radiotherapy given post-operatively reduces the risk of recurrence in the vaginal vault or elsewhere in the pelvis, but has no effect on distant secondaries, which most commonly appear in the lungs, and so the influence of radiation on overall survival is questionable.

Progestins are effective in the management of metastatic disease and between 35 and 40 per cent of women with lung or bone secondaries will gain a response; with disease at other sites this figure falls to about 20 per cent. There is some evidence for a dose response effect with high-dose progestogen therapy giving slightly better response rates. These results have encouraged the use of progestins as an adjuvant to surgery in early disease; retrospective analyses have suggested that this might be of value, but definitive proof from prospective randomised studies is still awaited.

Cytotoxic therapy is occasionally of value in metastatic disease, but because of the reduced toxicity of endocrine therapy the progestogens are usually the preferred first-line therapy.

Carcinoma of the Ovary

Ovarian cancer is the fifth commonest cancer in women and carries a high mortality as the disease is usually advanced by the time it is diagnosed: 60 per cent of patients having spread of tumour outside the pelvis at the time of presentation.

For the 20 to 25 per cent of women whose disease is limited to one or both ovaries, surgery, with a hysterectomy and bilateral salpingo-oophorectomy, is the treatment of choice giving a five-year survival of 60 to 70 per cent. For the more advanced stages of disease initial surgery is still mandatory as it has been shown that the greater the degree of removal, or debulking, of tumour then the better the overall survival. The value of giving radiotherapy following resection is uncertain. There have been claims that pelvic or total abdominal irradiation has improved survival, but there is considerable scepticism at these results.

Studies during the 1960s clearly demonstrated the sensitivity of advanced ovarian cancer to single drug chemotherapy with alkylating agents. Chlorambucil, melphalan and cyclophosphamide all gave response rates of 40 to 50 per cent with an average duration of about twelve months but there was no evidence of increased overall survival. During the 1970s various combination regimes were explored with the addition of other active agents such as doxorubicin and hexamethylmelamine. Although response rates were increased there was little, if any, change in five-year survival figures.

The introduction of cisplatinum in the early 1980s led to a further improvement in response rates and this drug and its later analogue, carbo-platin, are clearly the most active agents in ovarian cancer. Most recent combination schedules have included cisplatinum and response rates as high as 90 per cent have been seen in some studies in advanced disease. The effect on survival is mixed, however, as although there is no doubt that the median life-expectancy is increased by some 6 to 8 months as the result of the use of platinum compounds, the number of long-term survivors still alive at 5 years is similar to that seen with single agent alkylating therapy at about 5 per cent.

What then is the place of chemotherapy in the management of ovarian carcinoma? For very early disease, with growth limited to one ovary and no extension through the ovarian capsule, there is little to suggest that adjuvant chemotherapy will improve on the results of surgery alone. In advanced disease, where individual tumour deposits greater than 2cm in diameter remain after debulking surgery, chemotherapy is most unlikely to achieve a cure but aggressive treatment, using platinum-based regimes, will lead to a modest increase in survival and is indicated for younger patients in good general condition; for older or less well women single drug therapy with an alkylating agent may still achieve a temporary benefit. There remains a substantial group of patients whose stage of disease at presentation falls between these two extremes: those in whom tumour initially extended outside the ovary but after debulking surgery have either no macroscopic disease or minimal residual tumour (with individual deposits less than 2cm). It is very likely that aggressive chemotherapy increases short-term survival in these patients and may result in a small percentage of long-term survivors so platinum-based cytotoxic therapy is clearly indicated although clinical trials are still in progress to identify the optimum regime and to define precisely the benefits of such treatment.

The possible role for intraperitoneal chemotherapy in ovarian carcinomas was considered in Chapter 8.

Choriocarcinoma

Choriocarcinoma is a malignant tumour arising from the placenta. About once in every 2,000 pregnancies gross hypertrophy of the placenta occurs, resulting in the death of the foetus; this benign placental growth is termed a hydatidiform mole. In less than 10 per cent of cases remnants of this tumour will persist to form a true carcinoma of the chorion of the placenta. The persistant secretion of high levels of β-human chorionic gonadotrophin (hCG) is the key marker for the presence of such growths and the hCG level in the blood provides a sensitive measure of the response to treatment.

Despite its rarity, choriocarcinoma has an important place in the history of cancer chemotherapy in that it was the first solid tumour where cytotoxic treatment radically altered the prognosis and resulted in cure of previously incurable disease. Prior to cytotoxic therapy, treatment was by hysterectomy or irradiation and resulted in a 40 per cent cure rate for women with tumour confined to the uterus, whilst for those with metastatic disease death was invariable and rapid.

All women who present with hydatidiform moles in the UK today are followed up by serial hCG measurements. Those who develop choriocarcinoma are classified, on the basis of a number of prognostic variables (including age, parity, hCG level, site and size of metastases), as either low-, medium- or high-risk. Low-risk patients receive methotrexate and folinic acid, medium-risk patients receive a seven-drug combination made up of methotrexate, hydroxyurea, 6-mercaptopurine, actinomycin-D, and cyclophosphamide. The high-risk group receive a five-drug ...th 6-mercaptopurine and hydroxyurea being omitted from the above schedule, but with an increase in the dose of a number of the other agents.

As a result of these measures, cure rates today for low- and medium-risk patients are virtually 100 per cent and over 80 per cent in the high-risk group. In addition, hysterectomy no longer forms part of the management and so these young women retain their reproductive capacity.

Head and Neck Cancer

Head and neck cancers comprise a miscellaneous group of tumours which together account for about 3 per cent of all malignant disease. The majority of these lesions are squamous cell carcinomas arising from mucosal lining of the oral cavity or the upper respiratory and alimentary tracts. The rest of this discussion will be confined to these tumours.

The prognosis for squamous cell carcinoma in the head and neck varies considerably depending on the site of the lesion, over 90 per cent of carcinomas of the vermilion border of the lower lip are cured whilst the cure rate for carcinomas of the pyriform fossa is less than 5 per cent. Despite this variation in outlook the natural history of these tumours is similar in that they are locally invasive and spread to adjacent lymph nodes, distant metastases being a late and uncommon event. In head and neck cancer death is usually due to a failure to control local disease.

The treatment of choice for these lesions is surgery or radiotherapy or a combination of the two. By virtue of their localised nature even advanced lesions may be palliated by irradiation. Chemotherapy has been extensively used to try and control relapse after primary treatment and methotrexate has been the drug of choice. It has been given intravenously, orally and intra-arterially and often combined with leucovorin rescue in order that ultra-high doses might be given. Although the varied nature of the tumours makes assessment difficult, a greater than 50 per cent regression is seen in about 40 per cent of patients overall as a result of methotrexate therapy. The results of intra-arterial infusion show no advantage over intravenous therapy and as the former technique has considerable morbidity and mortality it has now largely been abandoned. Similarly, there is no clear evidence that high-dose therapy gives any better results than lower doses of methotrexate but some oncologists still use high-dose regimes.

Cisplatinum, bleomycin and 5-fluorouracil also have activity in head and neck cancer and many different multidrug regimes have been employed, cisplatinum and 5-fluorouracil being one of the most widely used combinations in recent years. It is quite clear that the use of such combinations improves response rates when compared to either methotrexate or cisplatinum used as single agents, although the precise figures vary considerably in different series. There is no evidence, however, that this improvement in response is reflected in any increase in survival and the value of such regimes remains controversial. In order to try and have an effect on survival times there have been numerous trials using chemotherapy as an adjuvant to primary surgery and/or radiotherapy and more recently neo-adjuvant therapy has also been evaluated. Although claims of a benefit have often been made from uncontrolled series there is, as yet, no evidence from any randomised trial of enhanced cure rates as a result of these efforts.

Malignant Melanoma

Skin cancers are extremely common, but the great majority of these are either basal cell carcinomas (rodent ulcers) or squamous cell carcinomas. Radiotherapy or surgery may be used to treat these lesions and result in cure in over 95 per cent of patients. Apart from the application of 5 per cent 5-fluorouracil cream to extremely superficial lesions cytotoxic therapy has no place in the management of these tumours. Malignant melanomas account for only 2 per cent of skin malignancies but they are aggressive cancers with a five-year survival rate of only 30 per cent. This poor prognosis, coupled with the many interesting clinical features of the disease, has given it an importance out of all proportion to its incidence.

Primary treatment consists of wide excision of the melanoma with skin grafting of the excision site. Local lymphatic spread is treated by surgery or radiotherapy. The treatment of disseminated disease relies on cytotoxic administration or the use of biological response modifiers. Unfortunately, the results of both these treatment modalities are generally disappointing. Almost all cytotoxic drugs have been tried in this condition and the great majority bring about responses in less than 10 per cent of patients. Dacarbazine and vindesine are the two most active single agents, with response rates approaching 20 per cent, but neither have any impact on increasing survival. Occasional responses have also been reported following the use of interferons. Combination chemotherapy has not made a significant contribution to management, although many regimes have been explored, and randomised studies of adjuvant therapy with various cytotoxic agents and biological response modifiers have proved consistently negative.

The role of regional chemotherapy in the management of malignant melanoma was discussed in Chapter 8.

Brain Tumours

The great majority of brain tumours in adults are astrocytomas and at the time of presentation these are generally advanced, poorly differentiated lesions, classified as glioblastoma multiforme. The outlook with such tumours is poor. These tumours very rarely metastasise and their lethal effect is due to direct infiltration and destruction of vital centres in the brain or a fatal increase in intracranial pressure due to associated inflammation and oedema. Treatment is, therefore, essentially local. Few lesions are resectable, however, and surgery alone results in a median survival of less than 3 months. It is now clear that the addition of radiotherapy improves the outlook but, even so, the median survival is only increased to between 6 and 12 months and only 5 to 10 per cent of patients are still alive after two years.

Cytotoxic therapy has been generally disappointing in these tumours, largely because of the inability of most drugs to cross the blood–brain barrier. One group of drugs, the nitrosoureas, do have high lipid solubility and, therefore, gain access to cerebral tissue and they have been extensively evaluated in these tumours. It is now clear that when used as single agent adjuvant therapy following initial surgery and irradiation, BCNU, CCNU and methyl-CCNU all have a small but statistically significant effect on increasing survival time. Overall, about 10 per cent more patients are alive at one year and five per cent more at two years as a result of chemotherapy. Clearly such a benefit is only marginal but there is no immediate prospect of improving on these results.

Corticosteroids, and in particular dexamethasone, are widely used to relieve symptoms due to progressive glioblastoma and are frequently effective for short periods of time. In the past, it has been suggested that this transient benefit might be evidence of a cytotoxic effect, but it is now generally considered to be the result of a reduction in the oedema and inflammation surrounding the tumour. This anti-inflammatory effect, although offering useful palliation, does not prolong survival.

Osteogenic Sarcoma

This is a rare tumour, only about 150 new cases appearing each year in the United Kingdom, but it is of great interest as the use of adjuvant chemotherapy in this condition has led initially to great optimism and subsequently to controversy. Survival data prepared in the early 1970s showed that at five years only 20 per cent of patients were still alive. More than 80 per cent of the tumours had apparently been localised at presentation but the great majority of these relapsed, usually with the appearance of lung secondaries, following initial surgery and radiotherapy. Non-randomised studies in the late 1970s used adjuvant chemotherapy, initially with high-dose methotrexate alone and subsequently with the addition of doxorubicin, and showed an apparent improvement in results with a prediction that 50 to 60 per cent of patients would be free of disease at five years. Other figures, produced at about the same time, suggested an alternative view, namely that the change in outlook was due to a change in the natural history of the disease and was independent of chemotherapy since survival appeared to be improving even in those who had no drug treatment.

To try and resolve this issue, a number of randomised studies have now been carried out. Although the results from a number of these series are now available there is still an element of confusion in that some negative results have been reported. The probability is, however, that these were due to inadequate cytotoxic dosage and most of the evidence does suggest that chemotherapy is of benefit and that adjuvant treatment, initially with high-dose methotrexate and doxorubicin and latterly with the addition of cisplatinum, has increased 5-year survival from 20 per cent to over 50 per cent in these patients. Most authorities would still consider, however, that such treatment should only be given in the context of a controlled clinical trial as important questions as to the optimum drug combination, dose and schedule remain to be answered. In particular, the value of neo-adjuvant therapy and its possible role in avoiding subsequent amputation is being carefully evaluated.

Soft Tissue Sarcomas

The soft tissue sarcomas are a varied group of tumours of mesenchymal origin. They include malignant fibrous histiocytomas, liposarcomas, adult rhabdomyosarcomas, synovial sarcomas, fibrosarcomas and leiomyosarcomas. Despite the heterogenous nature of these cancers, the prognosis appears to depend more on the size and histological grade of the primary lesion at the time of diagnosis rather than on its cell of origin. About 50 per cent of soft tissue sarcomas arise on the extremities.

After excision of the primary, even when this appears pathologically complete, local recurrence will occur in 40 to 80 per cent of cases. Post-operative radiotherapy reduces this figure to less than 20 per cent. Even with this combined treatment distant metastases, usually in the lungs, will develop in about half the patients (the risk varying from 25 per cent of those with low-grade tumours to 80 per cent in those with high-grade lesions).

Doxorubicin has proved the most effective single agent in metastatic disease with a response rate *averaging* 30 per cent, although this figure has varied enormously in different series. The most widely used combination regime has been CYVADIC (cylcophosphamide, vincristine, doxorubicin and dacarbazine); again response rates vary considerably in different reports, ranging from 10 to 50 per cent. More recently high-dose ifosfamide, with mesna, has given response rates of over 20 per cent and the combination of ifosfamide and doxorubicin is currently being evaluated. Although it is clear from these results that temporary tumour control may be achieved in advanced disease, there is no evidence that the use of chemotherapy actually increases survival.

There has been increasing interest in adjuvant cytotoxic therapy for soft tissue sarcomas over the last decade. A number of clinical trials using doxorubicin-based regimes have now been reported. Several series with small numbers of patients have claimed a survival advantage but in those studies randomising more than one hundred patients there has been no evidence of improved overall survival.

Bibliography

Chapter 1

Cellular growth and cancer formation, Iversen OH (1970) British Journal of Hospital Medicine, 3: 105–113
The cell cycle, Baserga R (1981) New England Journal of Medicine, 304: 453–459
Cell kinetics and cancer chemotherapy. Tannock IF in Fundamentals of Cancer Chemotherapy (Eds. Hellman K, Carter SK) McGraw Hill, New York, 1987, pp 7–19
Principles of cancer biology: kinetics of cellular proliferation. Hellman S, DeVita VT in Cancer: Principles and Practice of Oncology (Eds DeVita VT, Hellman S, Rosenberg S) JB Lipincott, Philadelphia, 1982, pp 73–79

Chapter 2

Chemotherapy. Lazlo J. Lucas VS, Stevenson D in Physician's Guide to Cancer Care Complications (Ed. Laszlo J) Marcel Dekker, New York, 1986, pp 61–146
Toxicity of chemotherapy. Perry MC, Yarbro JW (eds) Grune & Stratton, Florida, 1984
The acute toxicities of chemotherapy. Spiegel RJ (1981) Cancer Treatment Reviews, 8: 197–208
Fertility in long-term survivors of cancer. Byrne J, Mulvihill JJ, Myers MH (1987) New England Journal of Medicine, 317: 1315–1321
The effect of chemotherapy and radiotherapy on fertility and their prevention. Chapman RM, Sutcliffe S in Recent Advances in Clinical Oncology II (Eds. Williams CJ, Whitehouse JMA) Churchill Livingstone, 1986, pp 239–252
Second malignancies from adjuvant chemotherapy? Too soon to tell. Henderson IC, Gelman R (1987) Journal of Clinical Oncology, 5: 1135–1137

Chapter 3

Pharmacologic principles of cancer treatment. Chabner B (editor) WB Saunders, Philadelphia, 1982

Metabolism and action of anticancer drugs. Powis G, Prough RA (editors) Falmer Press, Philadelphia, 1986

Ifosfamide: pharmacology, safety and therapeutic potential. Brade WP, Herdrich K, Varini M (1985) Cancer Treatment Reviews, 12, 1–17

Hexamethylmelamine: a critical review of an active drug. Foster BJ, Harding BJ, Leyland-Jones B, Horth D (1986) Cancer Treatment Reviews, 13: 197–218

Epirubicin: a review of the pharmacology, clinical activity and adverse effects of an adriamycin analogue. Cersosimo RJ, Hong WK (1986) Journal of Clinical Oncology, 4: 425–439

Pharmacokinetics and metabolism of epidoxorubicin and doxorubicin in humans. Mross K et al (1988) Journal of Clinical Oncology, 6: 517–526

Progress in anthracycline therapy. Various authors (1987) Clinical Trials Journal, 24, Supplement 1: 1–250

Carboplatin: current status and future prospects. Canetta R, Bragman K, Smaldone L, Rosencweig M (1988) Cancer Treatment Reviews, 15: Supplement B: 17–32

Cancer chemotherapy: carboplatin v cisplatin. Anonymous (1987) Drug & Therapeutics Bulletin, 25: 67–68

Whither carboplatin? A replacement for or an alternative to cisplatin? Von Hoff D (1987) Journal of Clinical Oncology, 5: 169–171

Novantrone (mitozantrone). Cotter FE (1988) The British Journal of Clinical Practice, 42: 207–209

Mitozantrone. Anonymous (1986) Drug and Therapeutics Bulletin, 24: 71–72

Mitozantrone. Nathanson L (1984) Cancer Treatment Reviews, 11: 289–301

Amsacrine (AMSA). Isell BF (1980) Cancer Treatment Reviews, 7: 73–85

Chapter 4

Functional organisation of the hematopoietic stem cell compartment: implications for cancer and its therapy. Hellman S, Reincke U, Botnick L, Mauch P (1983) Journal of Clinical Oncology, 1: 277–284

High-dose methotrexate: a critical reappraisal. Ackland SP, Schilsky RL (1987) Journal of Clinical Oncology, 5; 2017–2031

Preoperative (neoadjuvant) chemotherapy. Recent Results in Cancer Research 103 Ragaz J, Band PR, Goldie JH (editors) Springer Verlag, Berlin 1986

Continuous infusion chemotherapy: a critical review. Vogelzang NJ (1984) Journal of Clinical Oncology, 2: 1289–1299

A rationale for the use of alternating non-cross resistant chemotherapy. Goldie JH, Goldman AJ (1982) Cancer Treatment Reports, 66: 439–449

Implications of dose intensity for clinical trials. Pater JL (editor) (1987) Seminars in Oncology, 14, Supplement 4: 1–44

Dose-response is alive and well. DeVita VT (1986) Journal of Clinical Oncology, 4: 1157–1159

The importance of dose intensity in chemotherapy of metastatic breast cancer. Hryniuk W, Bush H (1984) Journal of Clinical Oncology, 4: 1281–1288

Chapter 5

Prophylactic granulocyte transfusion during chemotherapy of acute nonlymphocytic leukemia. Winston DJ, Ho WG, Gale RP (1981) Annals of Internal Medicine, 94: 616–622

Platelet transfusion therapy. Anonymous (1987) Lancet, 2: 490–491

Broad spectrum antibacterial regimes for the seriously ill. Anonymous (1986) Drug and Therapeutics Bulletin, 24: 33–36

The use of anti-emetics during cancer chemotherapy. Allan SG (1986) Cancer Topics, 5: 126–127
Antiemetic therapy and cancer chemotherapy. Gralla RJ in Fundamentals of Cancer Chemo-
  therapy (Eds. Hellman K, Carter SK) McGraw Hill, New York, 1987, pp 387–396
Domperidone: an alternative to metoclopramide. Anonymous (1988) Drug and Therapeutic
  Bulletin, 26: 59–60
Etiology and treatment of chemotherapeutic agent extravasation injuries: a review. Rudolph R,
  Larson DL (1987) Journal of Clinical Oncology, 5: 116–126
Therapy of local toxicities caused by extravasation of cancer chemotherapeutic drugs. Ignoffo
  RJ, Friedman MA (1980) Cancer Treatment Reviews, 7: 17–27
Mesna – a short review. Shaw IC, Graham MI (1987) Cancer Treatment Reviews, 14: 67–86.

Chapter 6

Precautions for the safe handling of cytotoxic drugs. Guidance Note MS 21 from the Health &
  Safety Executive, HMSO, 1983
Handling of injectable antineoplastic agents. Knowles RS, Virden JE (1980) British Medical
  Journal, 281: 589–591
Regional policy for the safe handling of cytotoxic drugs. West Midlands Regional Health
  Authority, 1987
Preparation and administration of antineoplastic agents: risks and recommendations. Hillcoat
  BL, Levi J, Snyder R (1983) Australian Medical Journal, 1: 424–426

Chapter 7

Antitumor drug resistance. Fox BW, Fox M (editors) Springer Verlag, Berlin, 1984
Multidrug resistance. Moscow JA, Cowan KH (1988) Journal of the National Cancer Institute,
  80: 14–20
Multiple drug resistance in human cancer. Pastan I, Gottesman M (1987) New England Journal
  of Medicine, 316: 1388–1393
The cell membrane and drug resistance. Plumb JA, Kaye SB (1986) Cancer Topics, 6: 30–31

Chapter 8

Long term venous access. Peters JL, Belsham PA, Taylor BA, Watt-Smith S (1984) British
  Journal of Hospital Medicine, 32: 230–242
Home continuous infusion chemotherapy. Rowland CG (1985) The Practitioner, 229: 889–894
Vascular perfusion in cancer therapy. Recent Results in Cancer Research 86 Schwemmle K,
  Aigner K (editors). Springer Verlag, Berlin, 1983
Diagnosis and treatment of malignant pleural effusions. Fentiman IS (1987) Cancer Treatment
  Reviews, 14: 107–118
Malignant pleural effusions. Friedman MA, Slater F (1978) Cancer Treatment Reviews, 5: 49–66
Intraperitoneal chemotherapy: a review. Brenner DE (1986) Journal of Clinical Oncology, 4:
  1135–1147

Intraperitoneal antineoplastic agents for tumors principally confined to the peritoneal cavity. Markman M (1986) Cancer Treatment Reviews, 13: 219–242.

The biology and treatment of superficial bladder cancer. Torti FM, Lum BL (1984) Journal of Clinical Oncology, 2: 505–531

Effect of intravesical mitomycin-C on recurrence of newly diagnosed superficial bladder cancer. Tolbey DA, Hargreave TB, Smith PH, Williams JL et al (1988) British Medical Journal, 296: 1759–1761

Chapter 9

Antineoplastic agents and FDA regulations: square pegs for round holes. Wittes RE (1987) Cancer Treatment Reports, 71: 795–806

Drug development at the National Cancer Institute: a historical perspective. Zubrod CG in Fundamentals of Cancer Chemotherapy (Eds. Hellman S, Carter SK) McGraw Hill, New York, 1987, pp 101–110

Symposium on methodology and quality assurance in clinical trials. Various authors (1985) Cancer Treatment Reports, 69: 1039–1230

Anti-cancer drugs 5: Phase I trials. Calvert AH, Balmanno K (1987) Cancer Topics, 6: 51–52

Anti-cancer drugs 6: The design of phase II trials. Newlands E (1987) Cancer Topics, 6: 63–65

Anti-cancer drugs 7: Phase III and IV trials. Foster BJ (1987) Cancer Topics, 6: 87–89

Clinical evaluation of antitumour therapy Muggia FM, Rozencweig M (editors). Martinus Nijhoff, Boston, 1987

Illusion and reality: practical pitfalls in interpreting clinical trials. Glatstein E, Makuch RW (1984) Journal of Clinical Oncology, 2: 488–497

The effect of measuring error on the results of therapeutic trials in advanced cancer. Moertel CG, Hanley JA (1976) Cancer, 38: 388–398

Measurement of the quality of life after cancer treatment. Selby P (1985) British Journal of Hospital Medicine, 33: 266–271

Measuring and analysing quality of life in cancer clinical trials: a review. Fayers PM, Jones DR (1983) Statistics in Medicine, 2: 429–446

Chapter 10

Biological response modifiers. Pinsky CM (editor) (1986) Seminars in Oncology, 13: 131–258

Immunotherapy of cancer: the end of the beginning? Durant JR (1987) New England Journal of Medicine, 316: 938–940

Lymphokines. Dinarello C, Mier J (1987) New England Journal of Medicine 317: 940–945

Human interferon as a therapeutic agent: a decade passes. Merigan TC (1988) New England Journal of Medicine, 318: 1458–1460

Clinical overview of alpha interferon: studies and future directions. Spiegel RJ (1987) Cancer, 59: 626–631

Genes and cancer: a clinical perspective. Ellis M, Sikora K (1987) Journal of the Royal College of Physicians, 21: 122–128

Proto-oncogenes and human cancer. Slamon D (1987) New England Journal of Medicine, 317: 955–957

Tumour growth factors. Stroobant P (1986) Cancer Topics, 5: 128–129

Chapters 11 and 12

Endocrine therapy of breast cancer Cavalli F (editor) Springer Verlag, Berlin, 1986
The clinical biology of hormone responsive breast cancer. Epstein RJ (1988) Cancer Treatment
    Reviews, 15: 33–52
Breast cancer II. Bonadonna G (editor) (1987) Seminars in Oncology, 14: 1–83
Chemotherapy and hormonal therapy in combination. Hug V, Thomas H, Clark J (1988) Journal
    of Clinical Oncology, 6: 173–177
Advances in the management of hormone-responsive diseases. Various authors (1988) Seminars
    in Oncology, 15: Supplement 1: 1–78
Steroid receptors and clinical outcome in patients with adenocarcinoma of the endometrium.
    Ehrlich CE, Young PCM, Stehman FB et al (1988) American Journal of Obstetrics and
    Gynecology, 158: 796–807
Tamoxifen in breast cancer. Anonymous (1986) Drug and Therapeutics Bulletin, 24: 65–67
Aromatase inhibitors for treatment of breast cancer: current concepts and new perspectives.
    Santen RJ (1986) Breast Cancer Research and Treatment, 7 (supplement) S23–S25
Current status of high dose progestin treatment in advanced breast cancer. Mattson W (1983)
    Breast Cancer Research and Treatment, 3: 231–235
Glucocorticoid treatment for brain metastases and epidural spinal cord compression: a review.
    Weissman DE (1988) Journal of Clinical Oncology, 6: 543–551

Chapter 14

Cancer in children: clinical management Voute PA, Barrett A, Bloom HJG, Lemerle J,
    Neidhardt MK (editors). Springer Verlag, Berlin, 1986
Improvements in survival from childhood cancer: results of a population based survey over 30
    years. Birch JM, Marsden HB, Morris Jones PH, Blair V (1988) British Medical Journal, 296:
    1372–1376
Symposium on childhood cancer. Various authors (1986) Cancer, 58: 407–602

Chapter 15

Leukaemia. Whittaker JA, Delamore IW (editors) Blackwell Scientific Publications, Oxford,
    1987
Treatment of childhood acute lymphoblastic leukaemia. Anonymous (1988) Lancet, i: 683–685
Curing children of leukemia. Pinkel D (1987) Cancer, 59: 1683–1691
Acute lymphoblastic leukemia. Murphy SB (editor) (1985) Seminars in Oncology, 12: 79–195
Acute myeloid leukemia. Bloomfield CD (editor) (1987) Seminars in Oncology, 14: 357–468
Bone marrow transplantation for patients with chronic myeloid leukaemia. Mackinnon S,
    Goldman M (1988) British Journal of Hospital Medicine, 22: 226–230
Hodgkin's and non-Hodgkin's lymphomas: clinical assessment and treatment. Horwich A in
    Malignant lymphomas (Eds. Habeshaw JA, Lauder I) Churchill Livingstone, Edinburgh, 1988,
    pp 252–283
Curable cancers: Hodgkin's and non-Hodgkin's lymphomas. McElwain TJ (1984) British Journal
    of Hospital Medicine, 18; 10–19

ABVD versus MOPP: which is better? Rosenberg SA (1987) Journal of Clinical Oncology, 5: 7
MOPP after two decades. Rosenberg SA (1986) Journal of Clinical Oncology, 4: 1289–1290
Polycythaemia vera: an update. Berlin NI (editor) (1986) Seminars in Haematology, 23: 131–183
Plasma cell myeloma and the myeloma proteins. Farhangi M (editor) (1986) Seminars in Oncology, 13: 259–380
Management of multiple myeloma. Richards JDM, Singer CRJ, Tobias S (1987) British Journal of Hospital Medicine, 21: 437–442
Management of refractory myeloma: a review. Buzard AC, Durie BGM (1988) Journal of Clinical Oncology, 6: 889–905

Chapter 16

Lung cancer. Bunn P (editor) (1988) Seminars in Oncology, 15: 197–315
National lung cancer conference. Various authors (1987) British Journal of Cancer, 56: 881–900
Lung cancer: when to give chemotherapy. Anonymous (1988) Drug and Therapeutics Bulletin, 26: 29–30
Treatment of non-small cell lung cancer. Mulshine JL, Glatstein E, Ruckdeschel JC (1986) Journal of Clinical Oncology, 4: 1704–1715
Advanced non-small cell lung cancer: to treat or not to treat. Hansen HH (1987) Journal of Clinical Oncology, 5: 1711–1712
The medical management of breast cancer. Williams CJ, Buchanan RB. Castle House Publications, Tunbridge Wells, 1987
Adjuvant therapy for breast cancer. Henderson CI (1988) New England Journal of Medicine, 318: 443–444
Adjuvant tamoxifen in early breast cancer. Anonymous (1987) Lancet, 2: 191–192
Adjuvant tamoxifen for early breast cancer. Smith I (1988) British Journal of Cancer, 57: 527–528
Gastrointestinal oncology. Fielding JWL, Priestman TJ. Castle House Publications, Tunbridge Wells, 1986
Surgical adjuvant treatment of large bowel cancer. Moertel CG (1988) Journal of Clinical Oncology, 6: 934–936
Perspectives on treatment of large bowel cancer. Wittes RE (1988) Journal of the National Cancer Institute, 80: 5–7
Management of metastatic cancer of the prostate. Williams G (1988) Prescribers' Journal, 28: 43–48
Prostate cancer. Chisholm GD (1986) Cancer Topics, 6: 10–11
Management of metastatic prostatic carcinoma. Anonymous (1986) Drug & Therapeutics Bulletin, 24: 85–88
Renal-cell carcinoma. Harris DT, Maguire HC (editors) (1983) Seminars in Oncology, 10: 365–440
Chemotherapy of disseminated germ cell tumors. Einhorn LH (1987) Cancer, 60: 570–573
Testis cancer. Oliver RTD (1984) British Journal of Hospital Medicine, 18: 23–35
Clinical stage I carcinoma of the testis: a review. Fung CY, Garnick MB (1988) Journal of Clinical Oncology, 6: 734–750
The management of advanced testicular teratoma. Peckham MJ, Horwich A, Easton DF, Hendry WF (1988) British Journal of Urology, 62: 63–68
Pre-emptive (neo-adjuvant) intravenous chemotherapy for invasion bladder cancer. Raghaven D (1988) British Journal of Urology, 61: 1–8
Chemotherapy of urothelial tract tumors. Yagoda A (1987) Cancer, 60: 574–585
Common epithelial cancers of the ovary. Richardson GS, Scully RE, Nikrui N, Nelson JH (1985). New England Journal of Medicine, 312: 415–423 & 474–482
Controversy over combination chemotherapy in advanced ovarian cancer: what we learn from reports of matured data. Dembo AJ (1986) Journal of Clinical Oncology, 4: 1573–1576
Treating ovarian cancer. Burslem RW, Wilkinson PM (1986) British Medical Journal, 293: 972–973

Chemotherapy for advanced or recurrent gynecologic cancer. Thigpen T, Vance R, Lambuth B et al (1987) Cancer, 60: 2104–2116

Chemotherapy of gynecologic cancer (1984) Deppe G (editor) Alan R Liss, New York.

Developments in chemotherapy for medium and high-risk patients with gestational trophoblastic tumours (1979–1984). Newlands ES, Bagshawe KD, Begent RHJ, et al. (1986) British Journal of Obstetrics and Gynaecology, 93: 63–69

Head and neck cancer. Brady LW (editor) (1988) Seminars in Oncology, 15: 1–99

Why has so much chemotherapy done so little in head and neck cancer? Taylor SG (1987) Journal of Clinical Oncology, 5: 1–3

Brain tumours. Shapiro WR (editor) (1986) Seminars in Oncology, 13: 1–129

An overview of published results of randomised studies of nitrosoureas in primary high grade malignant glioma. Stenning SP, Freedman LS, Bleehen NM (1987) British Journal of Cancer, 56: 89–90

Malignant melanoma of the skin. Anonymous (1988). Drug & Therapeutics Bulletin, 26: 73–75

Osteosarcoma: fifteen years later. Goorin AM, Abelson HT, Frei E (1986) New England Journal of Medicine, 313: 1637–1642

Management of primary malignant bone tumours. Souhami RL (1987) Hospital Update, 13: 997–1009

Soft tissue sarcomas. Steward WP, Bramwell VHC (1986) Cancer Topics, 5: 138–140

The treatment of soft tissue sarcoma with focus on chemotherapy: a review. Pinedo HM, Verwij J (1986) Radiotherapy and Oncology, 5: 193–205

Subject Index

ABVD regime 66, 171, 172
Acrolein 30, 31, 79
Actinomyces 44
Actinomycin-D 19, 24, 44, 84, 92, 94, 101, 158, 160, 161, 192
Acute lymphoblastic leukaemia (ALL) 57, 90, 163–5
  B-cell 165
  common 165
  null-cell 165
  T-cell 165
  see also Leukaemia
Acute myeloid leukaemia (AML) 39, 50, 165–7
  see also Leukaemia
Adjuvant therapy 62–3, 103–4, 152, 180, 187, 191, 193
Adrenalectomy 182
Adrenocorticotrophic hormone (ACTH) 136–7
Adriamycin *see Doxorubicin*
Aldophosphamide 30
Alkylating agents 22, 27–35, 94, 102
  mode of action 28
  non-classical 46–8
  production of non-essential competitors 93
  see also under specific drugs
Allopurinol 40
Alopecia 20, 33, 43, 76–7
Aminoglutethimide 141–2, 182, 183
Aminopterin 36
Amsacrine 50, 84
Anaemia 74
Androgens 143, 182
Anoxia 62
Anthracenediones 49
  see also under specific drugs
Anthracycline antibiotics 42, 43–6, 94, 164
Anti-androgens 143, 186
Antibody formation 91
Anti-emetic agents 75

Antimetabolites 20, 27, 36–40
  mode of action 36–40
  see also under specific drugs
Antimicrobial chemotherapy 54
Antimitotic antibiotics 27, 42–6
  see also under specific drugs
Anti-oestrogens 139–41
  see also under specific drugs
Arabinoside 19
Ascites, control of 103
Asparaginase 50, 84, 91, 164
Astrocytomas 160, 193
Aziridines 34–5
  see also under specific drugs

B-lymphocytes 122
BACOP regime 174
Basal cell carcinomas 193
BCG 122
BCNU 35, 194
Biological response modifiers 121–8
Bladder carcinoma 187
Bladder irritation 105
Bleomycin 18, 19, 20, 24, 45, 69, 84, 102, 103, 171, 174, 192
Blood-brain barrier 90, 194
Bone marrow 3, 11, 17–18
Bone marrow suppression 31–5, 43, 46, 48, 49, 72
Bone marrow toxicity 72–4
Bone marrow transplantation 67, 73, 97, 161, 166
Bone tumours 161
Bowen's disease 106
Brain tumours 136, 160, 193–4
Breast cancer 57, 102, 136, 139–43, 179–84
  advanced 181–4
  early 179–81
  hormonal sensitivity in 131–3

Buserilin 144, 186
Busulphan 21, 34–5

Cachectin 125–6
Cancer treatment
    advantages and limitations of available
        treatment modalities 151–2
    objectives of 152–4
Cannabinoids 76
Carboplatin 18, 46, 84
Carboxyphosphamide 30
Carcino-embryonic antigen (CEA) 124
Carcinogenicity of cytotoxic drugs 23–6
Carcinoma. *See* under specific types and
        organs
Cardiac damage 31
Carmustine 84
Catecholamines 20
CCNU 18, 35, 160, 194
Cell cycle 7–9
    cytotoxic drugs, and 65–6
    kinetic implications 9–10
Cell growth 3, 4
Cell loss 10–11
Cell membrane 92
Cell population 3, 14, 17
Cell proliferation 15
Central nervous system (CNS) tumours 160
Cerebrospinal fluid (CSF) 105
Cervix, carcinoma 189
Chest pain 102
Childhood cancer 157–62
    relative incidence and survival 157
Chlorambucil 20–2, 24, 33, 190
CHOP regime 169, 174
Choriocarcinoma 36, 50, 191–2
Chromosomes 5, 6
Chronic lymphoid leukaemia (CLL) 168–9
    B-cell 168–9
    staging of 169
Chronic myeloid (granulocytic) leukaemia
        (CGL) 34, 50, 167–8
    see also Leukaemia
Cisplatinum 20, 24, 46, 76, 85, 104, 159, 161,
        162, 177, 178, 187–90, 192, 195
Clinical Trial Certificate (CTC) 107
Colorectal carcinoma. *See* Large bowel cancer
Combination chemotherapy 56–7, 174
    choice of drugs for 64–6
Complete response 113
Continuous infusion chemotherapy 68–9
COP regime 169
Corticosteroids 73, 77, 137, 182, 194
Corynebacterium parvum 102, 103, 122, 125
Cure, concept 53–4, 110–11
Cyclophosphamide 21, 22, 24, 30–2, 57, 67, 79,
        85, 103, 159–62, 164, 169, 174, 176, 177,
        180, 183, 190, 192, 195

Cyclosporin-A 95
Cyproterone acetate 143, 186
Cystitis 31, 105
Cytosine arabinoside 19, 24, 39, 85, 90, 93, 94,
        164, 165, 166
Cytotoxic drugs
    antagonism of action 78–9
    assessment criteria 110–11
    assessment of new 107–17
    carcinogenicity of 23–6
    cell-cycle phase-specific 90
    classification 27
    clinical evaluation 109–10
    cycle-specific 65
    development of 107–17
    effects on normal tissue 15–26
    health hazards 81
    management of side effects 71–9
    pharmacology of 27–51
    phase-specific 65
    precautions during preparation 82, 84–88
    precautions for administration 83, 84–88
    preclinical testing 107–8
    properties 15
    resistance to. *See* Drug resistance
    routine precautions against side effects 71–2
    scheduling of 61–4, 89–90
    toxicities 15–16
    treatment rationale 53–69
    see also under specific drugs
CYVADIC regime 195

Dacarbazine 20, 48, 85, 116, 159, 171, 193, 195
Daunorubicin 42, 43, 85, 92, 164, 166
Dexamethasone 76, 194
Dianhydrogalactitol 35
Diaries 116
Dibromodulcitol 35
Diethyl stilboestrol 142
Differentiated cells 17, 18
Dimethanesulphonates 34–5
    see also under specific drugs
DNA 25
DNA chain 6, 7, 29, 39, 43–5, 94
DNA complex 7
DNA cross-linkages 47
DNA duplication 7
DNA formation 39
DNA replication 29
DNA synthesis 7–9, 43, 44, 50
Dopamine 20
Doxorubicin 18–20, 24, 42, 43, 69, 86, 92,
        102–5, 159–62, 169, 171, 174, 177, 183,
        184, 187, 195
Drostanolone propionate 143
Drug access 62, 97–8
Drug activation 92–3
Drug administration 28

alternative methods of 97–106
central venous access 97–8
intra-arterial therapy 98–102
intraperitoneal therapy 103–4
intrapleural therapy 102
intrathecal therapy 105–6
intravesical therapy 104–5
precautions for 83, 84–88
timing 61–2
topical therapy 106
Drug antagonism 91
Drug deactivation 92
Drug dosage 27–8, 66–8
Drug resistance 62, 89–95
cellular factors causing 91–4
cross resistance 95
general factors 89–90
increased production of target molecule 93
prevention of 94–5
summary of 94
Durabolin 143

Emesis 74
Endocrine drugs 139–147
Endocrine therapy 131–7, 181–3, 190
Endometrial adenocarcinomas 189–90
Endometrial carcinoma 134–5
Enkephalin 20
Enzyme specificity 93
Enzyme therapy 50
Epipodophyllotoxins 49
see also under specific drugs
Epirubicin 43, 44, 86, 184
Epoxides 35
see also under specific drugs
Erythroplasia of Queyrat 106
Ethinyl oestradiol 142
Etoposide 20, 49, 86, 92, 94, 159, 162, 175, 177, 178, 192
Ewing's sarcoma 161–2
Extravasation 77–8

FAM regime 184
Fertility
female 23
male 22
α-Feta protein 188
5-Fluorouracil 19, 24, 38–9, 57, 67, 69, 86, 91, 93, 94, 101, 104, 106, 180, 183–5, 192, 193
Flutamide 143, 186
Folic acid 36
Follicle stimulating hormone (FSH) 139, 144
Fractional cell kill 55–6

Gastrointestinal cancer 45, 104, 153–5, 184–5
Gastrointestinal disturbance 48

Gastrointestinal epithelium 19
Gastrointestinal toxicity 31
Gastrointestinal tract 19–20
Genitourinary cancer 185–7
Glioblastoma multiforme 194
Glucocorticoids 136–7, 146–7
Goserilin acetate 144, 186
Graft-versus-host disease 166
Growth factor receptors (GFR) 132
Growth factors 127–8
Gynaecological cancer 189–92

Haematological cancers 163–76
Haemorrhagic cystitis 31, 79
Hair loss. See Alopecia
Hairy-cell leukaemia 169
Hallucinatory side effects 76
Head and neck cancer 99–100, 192–3
Health and Safety Executive 81
Hepatic metastases 100–1
Hexamethylmelamine 34
Hodgkin's disease 22, 24, 25, 30, 42, 48, 57, 68, 163, 169–72
staging of 170
see also Lymphoma
Honvan 142
5HT$_3$-receptors 19, 76
Human chorionic gonadotrophin (hCG) 188, 191
Hydrea 49–50
Hydrocortisone 165
4-Hydroxycyclophosphamide 30, 31
17β-Hydroxysteroid dehydrogenase 145
5-Hydroxytryptamine (serotonin) 19
Hydroxyurea 49–50, 175, 192
Hyperkeratosis 106
Hyperthermia 101
Hypophysectomy 182
Hypoxia 62

Ifosfamide 20, 31–3, 69, 72, 79, 86, 160–2, 178
Immunosuppression 26
Immunotherapy 121–2
Interferons 124–5, 135, 174
Interleukin-2 125
Intermittent chemotherapy 57–61
Intra-arterial therapy 98–102
Intraperitoneal therapy 103–4
Intrapleural therapy 102
Intrathecal therapy 105–6
Intravesical therapy 104–5

Karnofsky index 114–15
Kidney tumours 186

Large bowel cancer 67, 155
Leucopenia 49–50, 72–3
Leucovorin 67, 78–9, 100
Leukaemia 24, 25, 36, 40, 55, 62, 77, 97, 136,
    137, 163
  see also under specific diseases
Leuprolide 144
Levamisole 122
Leydig cells 22
Linear analogue self-assessment 115
Liver metastases 181
Lorazepam 76
Lung cancer 102, 177–8
  non-small cell 178
  small cell 177
Luteinising hormone (LH) 144
Luteinising hormone releasing hormone
    (LHRH) 134, 144, 186
Lymphokines 124–6
Lymphomas 24, 25, 30, 40, 62, 95, 136, 137,
    163
  see also Hodgkin's disease; Non-Hodgkin's
    lymphoma (NHL)

Malignant carcinoid tumour 185
Malignant melanoma 42, 101, 193
Medroxyprogesterone acetate 145, 183
Medulloblastomas 160
Megestrol acetate 145
Melphalan 18, 24, 33, 86, 176, 180, 184, 190
mer-BCG 122
6-Mercaptopurine 40, 92–5, 164, 192
Mesna 31, 32, 79
Metastatic disease 152, 159, 162, 180, 186, 187,
    190, 191
Methionine 20
Methotrexate 19, 21, 24, 36–8, 57, 78, 87,
    90–2, 94, 99, 104, 105, 164, 165, 175,
    180, 183, 187, 192, 195
Methyl-CCNU 35, 185, 194
Metoclopramide 75–6
Micrometastases 64, 152, 180
Minimal response 114
Mithramycin 45–6, 87, 92, 94
Mitomycin-C 20, 44–5, 72, 87, 104, 105, 178,
    184, 187
Mitosis 4–5
Mitozantrone 18, 49, 72, 87, 104, 184
MOF regime 185
Monoamine oxidase inhibitors 48
Monoclonal antibodies 122–4
MOPP regime 66, 171, 172
Multiple myeloma 77, 163, 176
Mustard gas 28
Mustine hydrochloride 29–30
Mycosis fungoides 106
Myelofibrosis 34
Myeloma 25

Myelosuppression 72
Myxoedema 136

Nausea 19–20, 74–6
Neo-adjuvant therapy 63, 159, 187, 195
Neuroblastoma 159–60
New Drug Approval (NDA) 107, 116
Nitrogen mustard 20, 24, 28–30, 57, 87, 102,
    103, 171
Nitrogen mustards 29–33
  see also under specific drugs
Nitrosoureas 24, 35, 72, 175, 184, 194
  see also under specific drugs
Nomograms 28
Non-anthracycline antibiotics 44–6
Non-Hodgkin's lymphoma (NHL) 163, 172–5
  classification of 173
  lymphoblastic 175
  treatment and survival in 174
Nucleic acids 5–7

Oestrogen receptors 132, 139
  clinical correlations 133
Oestrogen therapy 142, 182, 183
Oncogenes 126–7
Orchidectomy 189
Osteogenic sarcoma 194–5
Ovarian ablation 182
Ovarian cancer 33, 102, 104, 190–1
Ovary 23

Palliation 114–16
Papillary carcinomas 136
Partial response 113–14
Pericarditis-myocarditis syndrome 43
Personal cure 111
Pharmorubicin see Epirubicin
Phenothiazines 74, 76
Phosphoramide mustard 30
Phosphorylated methylstilboestrol 142
Phytohaemagglutinin 125
Placenta 191
Polycythaemia vera 34, 50, 163, 175
Prednisolone 164, 171
Prednisone 57, 169, 174
Pregnancy 21–2
Probenecid 105
Procarbazine 24, 48, 57, 72, 171
Product Licence application 107, 116
Progesterone receptors 132
Progestogens 144–5, 182, 190
Progression 114
Prostaglandins 20
Prostatic carcinoma 134, 141, 142, 185–6
Protein synthesis 44
Pulmonary toxicity 45

Quinacrine 102

Radiotherapy 152
Recruitment 56
Red blood cells 3, 17
Refractory malignant hypercalcaemia 46
Regional chemotherapy 101
Relapse-free survival 112
Renal cell carcinoma 135, 186–7
Reserpine 95
Respiratory insufficiency 35
Response criteria 113
Resting cells 11–13
Retinoblastoma 162
Rhabdomyosarcoma 160–1
RNA synthesis 43, 44
Rodent ulcers 193

Screening systems 108
Seminomas 189
Side effects, management of 71–9
Single-agent therapy 54–5, 174
Skin cancer 106, 193
    see also Malignant melanoma
Skin pigmentation 35
Skin toxicity 20–1, 45
Sodium bicarbonate 77
Soft tissue sarcomas 101, 195–6
Solid tumours 177–96
Spermatogenesis 22
Statistical cure 111
Stem cells, 11, 12, 17, 18
Steroid synthesis, inhibitors of 141–2
Streptomyces 42
Streptomyces caespitosus 44
Streptomyces verticillis 45
Streptozotocin 35
Sulphur mustard 28
Surgical treatment 151–2
Survival by response 112–13
Survival duration 111–12

Tamoxifen 95, 139–41, 181, 182
Tamoxifen-withdrawal response 141

Teniposide 49, 92, 94
Teratogenic effects 21
Testicular cancer 45, 68, 188–9
Testis 22
Tetracycline 102
6-Thioguanine 40, 93–5, 166
Thiotepa 24, 34, 87, 102–5
Thrombocythaemia 34
Thrombocytopenia 46, 48, 73–4
Thymosin 122
Thyroid gland carcinoma 136
Thyroid stimulating hormone (TSH) 136
Topical therapy 106
Triethylene thiophosphoramide 34
Tumour cells 12–14
Tumour control 103–4
Tumour doubling time 13
Tumour growth 3–14
    natural history 13–14
Tumour growth fraction 62
Tumour growth rate 54
Tumour necrosis factor (TNF) 125–6
Tumour regression and cure 53–4

Unborn child 21–2

VAC regime 177–178
Verapamil 95
Verbal rating scales 115
Vinblastine 42, 88, 171, 187
Vinca alkaloids 20, 21, 24, 27, 41–2, 69, 92, 94
    mode of action 41–2
    see also under specific drugs
Vinca rosea 41
Vincristine 41–2, 57, 88, 159–62, 164, 169, 171,
    174, 177, 185, 187, 192, 195
Vindesine 42, 88, 178, 193
Visual rating scales 115
Vomiting 19–20, 74–6

White blood corpuscles 17
Wilms' tumour 158–9

Xanthine oxidase 40